T0319093

CLINICAL MANAGEMENT OF ACUTE SKIN TRAUMA

CLINICAL MANAGEMENT OF ACUTE SKIN TRAUMA

JOEL W. BEAM

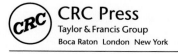

CRC Press
Taylor & Francis Group
Boca Raton London New York

CRC Press is an imprint of the
Taylor & Francis Group, an **informa** business

Designed cover image: Tinhouse Design

First published 2025
by CRC Press
2385 NW Executive Center Drive, Suite 320, Boca Raton FL 33431

and by CRC Press
4 Park Square, Milton Park, Abingdon, Oxon, OX14 4RN

CRC Press is an imprint of Taylor & Francis Group, LLC

© 2025 Taylor & Francis Group, LLC

ISBN: 9781638220664 (pbk)
ISBN: 9781003523055 (ebk)

DOI: 10.1201/9781003523055

Typeset in Minion Pro
by codeMantra

DEDICATION

To my parents, as your memories and spirit carry me daily.
To athletes, patients, students, and colleagues, thank you for the inspiration and support.

CONTENTS

ACKNOWLEDGMENTS

The development of a project such as this requires contributions of time, patience, expertise, and effort from many individuals. The concept of the textbook began with a conversation with Brien Cummings at SLACK Incorporated. I thank Brien for his vision and the opportunity to develop the textbook. Also at SLACK, thanks to Kayla Whittle who came on board to see the project to completion. I extend special gratitude to the contributing authors, Bernadette Buckley, PhD, LAT, ATC and Mario Ciocca, MD. Bernadette has been involved with me in the wound management journey from the beginning, providing vision and support in the research and scholarly projects. Completion of these projects would not have been possible without her assistance. Dr. Ciocca offered his knowledge and clinical expertise in preparing the infections and adverse reactions chapter, essential components in the management of acute skin trauma. The photographs and illustrations were made possible through the efforts of local athletic trainers, contributing authors, and University of North Florida Clinical and Applied Movement Sciences Department students and colleagues and the University of North Florida Center for Instruction and Research Technology (CIRT). At CIRT, Shelby Scanlon guided photo shoots, Brenna Smith created illustrations, and Andy Rush designed a web page for photograph submission. I would like to thank each of them for their support. Special thanks to Michael Boyles at CIRT for his creativity and proficiency in the final design of the photographs and illustrations. These contributions play a significant role in the presentation of the chapters.

ABOUT THE AUTHOR

Joel W. Beam, EdD, LAT, ATC is a professor and the chair of the Department of Clinical and Applied Movement Sciences in the Brooks College of Health at the University of North Florida (UNF) in Jacksonville, Florida. He also teaches within the Master of Science in Athletic Training Program at UNF. His interest in athletic training began in junior high as a student athletic trainer and continued through high school. Dr. Beam received his BS degree from East Carolina University in Greenville, North Carolina; his MEd from Clemson University in Clemson, South Carolina; and his EdD from UNF. He has 29 years of experience as an athletic trainer at the intercollegiate level through positions at 4 universities. Dr. Beam has taught athletic training courses at the university level for over 30 years and has held previous program director and clinical coordinator positions at UNF. His research focuses on the effectiveness of occlusive dressings on healing rates of standardized abrasions and the implementation of evidence-based acute skin trauma interventions into clinical practice. He has authored book chapters and manuscripts and given numerous presentations at international and national conferences and symposiums regarding acute skin trauma. Dr. Beam has also authored the textbook *Orthopedic Taping, Wrapping, Bracing, and Padding*.

CONTRIBUTING AUTHORS

Bernadette Buckley, PhD, LAT, ATC (Chapter 3)
University of North Florida
Jacksonville, Florida

Mario Ciocca, MD (Chapter 7)
University of North Carolina
Chapel Hill, North Carolina

INTRODUCTION

Trauma and subsequent injury to the skin are frequent with participation in athletic, recreational, and work activities. Various mechanisms of injury can produce abrasions, avulsions, blisters, lacerations, punctures, and traumatic and postoperative incisions. Proper management of these injuries is critical to creating an optimal environment to promote healing and lessen the risk of infection and adverse reactions. Wound management techniques have evolved over the last 60 years. However, ritualistic interventions and techniques continue in clinical practice today. Techniques such as cleansing the wound daily with topical antiseptics, using dressings that promote desiccation of the wound and formation of eschar, performing dressing changes without regard to the progression of healing, and leaving attached necrotic tissue to the periwound tissue to protect the wound can increase the risk of adverse reactions. During the 1960s, the discovery of a moist wound environment with occlusion of the wound challenged many time-honored practices. These investigations and other researchers examining cleansing, debridement, and dressing interventions transformed the approach to the management of acute skin trauma.

The paradigm of evidence-based medicine guides appropriate management of acute skin trauma, and implementation into clinical decision-making and practice can enhance the delivery of health care services to patients. The overall goal of *Clinical Management of Acute Skin Trauma* is to facilitate learning of the knowledge, skills, and clinical abilities required to manage acute skin trauma effectively. The text is intended for professional athletic training students, practicing athletic trainers, and other health care professionals responsible for acute wound care. Among students, the text can first be used in the didactic setting and then taken to the clinical setting for skill development. The material in the text covers the Board of Certification's Practice Analysis and the Commission on Accreditation of Athletic Training Education Curricular Content Standards related to the management of acute skin trauma. Students should have a general knowledge of human and skin anatomy, wound healing, and the assessment process to integrate the material in the chapters. Interventions can be introduced and practiced in didactic labs with wound models to provide real-world experiences. Among practicing athletic trainers and other health care professionals, the text can serve as a practical resource guide for evidence-based practice. For others, the text introduces evidence-based skin trauma management guidelines for implementation into current practice.

The chapters focus on individual components and interventions for the holistic management of acute skin trauma. Chapter 1 provides information on the types, etiology, assessment, clinical presentation, and initial management of acute skin trauma. Chapter 2 presents infection control guidelines and techniques for facilities and management plans and recommended wound management supplies for facilities and kits. Chapter 3 includes cleansing, Chapter 4 debridement, and Chapter 5 dressings for acute wounds. These chapters explain and illustrate evidence-based interventions and include the techniques' goals and objectives, indications, contraindications, and procedures. The selection and application factors to consider for patient management plans and summaries of the evidence are also presented. Chapter 6 discusses patient monitoring and reassessment and the role of patient education and adherence in the management plan. Chapter 7 explains the causes, clinical features, treatment, and prevention of infection and adverse reactions. Chapter 8 includes scenarios to allow students and clinicians the opportunity to bring together individual chapters, interventions, and factors to develop and revise management plans for patients. Several appendices are used to enhance the material for the reader. Appendix A presents an overview of wound closure with sutures and staples. Common suture and staple techniques are illustrated. Appendix B contains a wound care infographic that can be used for athlete, parent, and guardian education. Appendix C includes a clinical application table summarizing cleansing, debridement, and dressing techniques based on wound type. This table allows athletic training students and certified athletic trainers to carry the guide in athletic training kits and bags in clinical practice settings.

Clinical Management of Acute Skin Trauma will comprehensively guide the reader from the initial injury assessment through complete wound healing using evidence-based practice techniques for the management of acute skin trauma. Management considerations based on wound characteristics; patient needs and activity levels; financial, physical, and personnel resources; various sports, recreational, and work settings; and governing regulations will assist in the development of best-practice, evidence-based clinical applications. The use of color photographs throughout the chapters, step-by-step procedures of intervention techniques, and evidence summaries from the literature and clinical expertise plays an integral role in enhancing the presentation and learning of the material.

1

CLINICAL PRESENTATION AND ASSESSMENT

Acute skin trauma can result in varying levels of damage to the epidermis, dermis, or subcutaneous tissues. These injuries can result in superficial insult to the epidermis with no effect on athletic or work activities; other injuries may extend into the subcutaneous tissues and require referral for advanced cleansing, debridement, and wound closure. Appropriate assessment of patients with acute skin injury is critical to guide interventions, promote healing, and lessen the risk of complications. This chapter addresses the types, etiology, clinical presentation, assessment, clinical decision-making, and initial management of acute skin wounds.

ACUTE SKIN TRAUMA

The skin is the largest organ of the body and is composed of 3 layers: the epidermis, dermis, and subcutaneous tissue (Figure 1-1). Skin functions to provide mechanical support, structure, thermoregulation, and protection, serving as a physical barrier against trauma, external forces, and microorganisms. It undergoes daily assault from shear and tensile loads and forces during athletic, recreational, and work activities, often resulting in an open wound. Acute skin trauma is a disruption of the integrity of the epidermis, dermis, or subcutaneous tissues (or a combination of these

DOI: 10.1201/9781003523055-1

Figure 1-1. The layers of the skin.

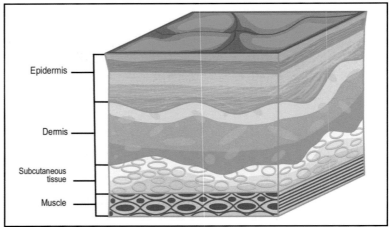

layers).[1] Disruption in the integrity of the epidermis, dermis, or subcutaneous tissues can compromise the protective functions of the skin and result in bacterial contamination, infection, and the development of other adverse reactions. Acute wounds progress through an orderly reparative process of inflammation, proliferation, and remodeling regardless of treatment, typically within 4 to 6 weeks, resulting in the restoration of anatomical and functional integrity.[2-5] The inflammatory stage initiates with platelet aggregation and the development of a fibrin clot followed by hemostasis. An inflammatory response is produced to cleanse the wound and prepare an environment for tissue repair. This response is characterized by **erythema**, swelling, warmth, and pain. The proliferation stage begins within hours after injury and results in re-epithelization of the wound and the formation of a new extracellular matrix. The final remodeling stage begins around the second week of healing and produces wound contraction, compaction, and strengthening. Healing tissues will continue to remodel and strengthen over the next few months. Appropriate cleansing, debridement, and dressing techniques can enhance the rates of healing and lessen the risk of adverse reactions.

TYPES OF ACUTE SKIN TRAUMA

The most common acute wounds include traumatic abrasions, avulsions, blisters, lacerations, punctures, and traumatic and postoperative incisions. Acute skin trauma occurs through intentional or unintentional external shear and tensile forces and tensile loads. Intentional trauma is a break or tear in the skin during a surgical procedure (eg, a postoperative incision). Unintentional trauma is a break or tear caused by an external, accidental mechanism (eg, a traumatic laceration). Trauma and subsequent injury can result from a single or repeated exposure to forces and loads. The clinical presentation is determined by the severity of the trauma and resultant tissue damage.[1,6] Superficial-thickness wounds involve injury to the superficial epidermis. Partial-thickness wounds extend through the epidermis and into part of the superficial dermis, and full-thickness wounds extend through the epidermis and dermis and into the subcutaneous adipose tissue.

Abrasions result from shear forces against a rough surface, typically in one direction.[7,8] They are common to the upper and lower extremities from contact with concrete, dirt, and artificial playing surfaces. Abrasions present with capillary bleeding, erythema of the **periwound tissue**, and possible contamination of the wound bed with debris (eg, sand, grass, dirt, or asphalt)[8] (Figure 1-2). Avulsions can result from tensile loads and result in skin and tissue failure.[7,8] These wounds may occur from violent contact with field or court structures (eg, a soccer goal) or protective equipment (eg, a helmet). They present with partial or complete separation of skin and tissue from its normal

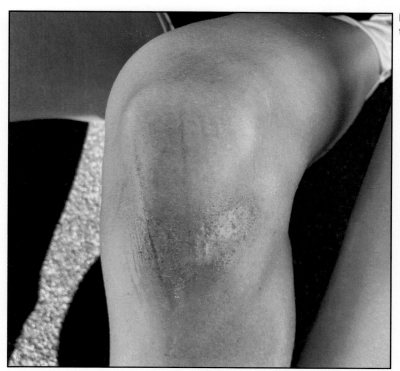

Figure 1-2. An abrasion on the anterior knee.

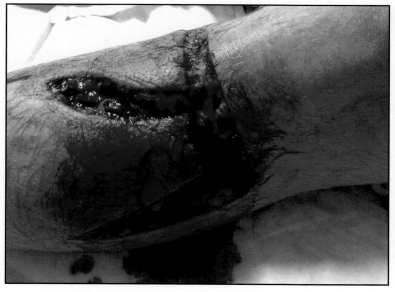

Figure 1-3. An avulsion on the anterior lower leg.

anatomical structure, venous or arterial bleeding, trauma to underlying tissues and structures, and contamination of skin and tissue flaps.[7,8] Completely avulsed tissue with debris can also result[7,8] (Figure 1-3). Blisters result from repeated unidirectional or multidirectional shear forces on moist skin.[8] These wounds are common to the feet and hands from contact with shoes and equipment. Blisters present with a collection of extracellular fluid trapped between the epidermis and dermis at the area of friction, erythema, and possible external hemorrhage and contamination.[8] Closed blisters

Figure 1-4. A closed blister on the plantar forefoot.

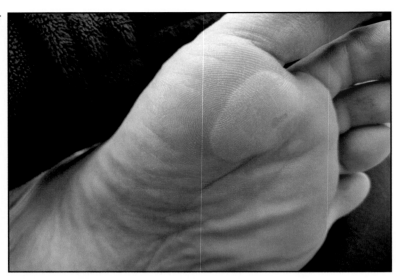

Figure 1-5. An open blister on the medial, posterior calcaneus.

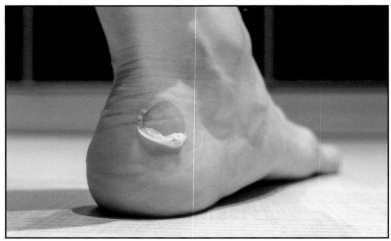

appear with a fluid-filled sac of varying size and erythema of the friction site and periwound tissue[8] (Figure 1-4). Open blisters appear as an acute wound with a **necrotic** flap or roof of the skin attached to the border of the drained sac, erythema of the periwound tissue, possible capillary bleeding, and contamination with debris (Figure 1-5). The flap or roof of the skin can be removed entirely from the blister margins at the assessment. Lacerations result from tension and shear forces, producing an irregular tear in the skin and tissue.[7,8] These wounds present with an irregular or jagged tear in the skin, venous or arterial bleeding, possible trauma to underlying structures, and contamination with debris[8] (Figure 1-6). Punctures result from penetrating tensile forces and loads from a cylindrical, sharp object.[8] These wounds present as a tear or cavity in the skin, with a possible embedded object in the wound, venous or arterial bleeding, possible trauma to the underlying structures, and contamination with debris and foreign bodies (Figure 1-7). Incisions result from sharp tensile forces, resulting in a clean tear in the skin.[7,8] They present with a regular or clean tear in the skin, venous or arterial bleeding, possible trauma to underlying structures, and contamination with debris[8] (Figure 1-8). Incisions, lacerations, and punctures can also result from contact with improperly maintained protective equipment (eg, exposed metal) and athletic structures (eg, bleachers and benches).

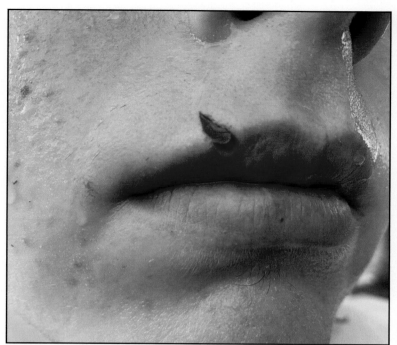

Figure 1-6. A laceration on the upper lip.

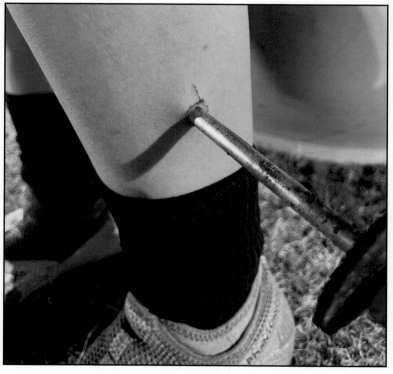

Figure 1-7. A puncture on the lateral lower leg caused by a soccer training pole.

Figure 1-8. An incision on the palmar fifth finger.

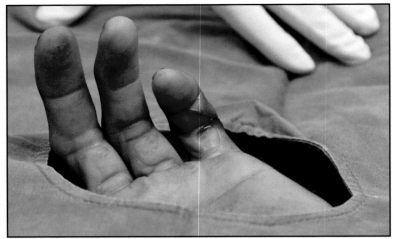

ASSESSMENT

Assessment of skin trauma, like all acute injuries, is performed through primary and secondary surveys of the patient. The primary survey assesses the cardiovascular and respiratory systems, head and cervical spine, profuse or uncontrolled bleeding, open or closed fractures, dislocations, and nerve injury to identify emergent conditions and guide further assessment and appropriate emergency treatment.[9] Additional guidelines for a primary survey and emergency treatment are described elsewhere. This section focuses on the secondary survey in the assessment of acute wounds.

Assessment of skin trauma typically occurs directly after injury; however, some patients delay seeking medical attention until athletic or work activity levels are affected by adverse reactions. The assessment goals are to determine a clinical diagnosis, identify patient factors that may affect healing, and develop treatment interventions including possible referrals. In the athletic setting, immediate postinjury assessments are often conducted on the field or court during practices and competitions, including whether a patient can safely return to play in a timely manner. Documentation of the assessment findings is critical for the clinical decision-making process and care of the patient. Chapter 2 discusses infection control guidelines, environmental considerations, and supplies needed for the assessment and management of acute skin trauma.

With most acute skin trauma injuries, the patient is ambulatory and conscious, and a secondary survey can be performed without complications.[7] The assessment is performed in a systematic or overlapping manner based on the clinician's knowledge of the patient. For example, access to and knowledge of the patient's prior medical history and records in the athletic setting can provide much of this information. The secondary survey should include a history, inspection, palpation, muscle and joint testing, neurologic and vascular assessments, and systems review as warranted.[9] The history consists of open-ended questions of demographics, past medical history, and present injury history. Questions regarding age, occupation, activity level, lifestyle, previous injury to the area and past treatment or surgery, occurrence of complications, and outcomes provide a baseline for treatment of the current injury. For example, a patient working in a hot, humid warehouse will require a wound dressing that will remain adherent in this environment. A patient traveling out of town for business during the week may need a dressing that can remain on the wound bed for longer periods until the next reassessment and education about dressing wear. A patient with a history of delayed healing from previous wounds may benefit from a referral to determine the causative factor(s). Clinicians should also obtain a health history of comorbid illnesses and conditions, current medications taken, status of tetanus prophylaxis vaccination, and allergies to materials used to treat acute wounds to lessen the risk of adverse reactions. The use of anti-inflammatory medications may produce a delay in healing. Sensitivity to topical antimicrobial creams and ointments, dressing adhesives, and occlusion of the skin with dressings can also result in adverse reactions.

A history of the present injury includes the mechanism of injury, time of injury, location and type of pain, presence of numbness or tingling, and sensations or sounds heard during the trauma and can indicate the level of tissue damage and associated trauma.[7] The mechanism and setting (eg, an athletic field or automotive factory) of the injury can determine the extent of contamination of the wound with debris and bacteria, tissue involvement, and possible associated trauma.[4] For example, a forearm abrasion sustained from sliding on a baseball dirt infield will likely be contaminated with small pieces of dirt and clay. A contusion to the forearm is also possible. The mechanism, setting, and time of injury can also predict the level of bacteria in the wound and the potential for infection.[10] Wounds that are associated with fracture, visibly contaminated, or deep; wounds with exposure of deep structures; wounds that are **stellate** or contain foreign debris; and delayed treatment of wounds can increase the risk of infection. The type and location of pain associated with acute wounds are commonly described as a stinging or sharp sensation localized to the damaged tissue or body area. Pain radiating, referred, deep, or associated with movement can indicate secondary trauma to other structures, and further assessment is required. Documentation of pain levels with visual analog or numeric rating scales can be performed. Numbness or tingling in an extremity can indicate nerve pathology and associated trauma. Sensations and sounds can be associated with fractures, strains, sprains, dislocations, and subluxations. In situations with delayed reporting of the wound, clinicians should obtain past treatment from the patient. Clinicians should ask if cleansing, debridement, or dressing interventions have been performed and what materials were used. The patient should also be asked if the wound has changed since the injury. How has the initial pain changed? How has the drainage from the wound changed? Has the wound bed dried and become painful? The patient's answers to these questions assist the clinician in determining which specific techniques, if any, have been performed.

A bilateral inspection of the patient requires the assessment of the wound location, length, width, and depth; the type and color of tissue in the wound bed; the type and amount of hemorrhage or **exudate**; the condition of the periwound tissue; swelling and deformity of the surrounding soft tissue; and the presence of debris in the wound.[11,12] Irrigation of the wound bed and periwound tissue with normal saline or **potable tap water** (without the presence of exposed bone or tendon)[1] may be required to identify tissue damage and the structures involved. The location, length, width, and depth can indicate the extent of the trauma, the type of wound, and tissue damage. The wound location, length, and width can impact the amount of skin tension and tissue approximation of the wound and determine dressing and closure methods. Deep wounds with exposed bone, tendon, or ligament structures should be referred for advanced cleansing, debridement, and closure.[12] The measurement of acute wounds through direct measurement, tracings, or photography is rarely performed based on the predictable healing progression with appropriate management techniques. The wound bed tissue type and color reveal the status of the wound and tissue viability (Table 1-1 and Figures 1-9 to 1-12). The immediate postinjury inspection typically reveals viable granulation tissue with varying amounts of contamination with debris. Based on the length of time from the injury, a delayed inspection may reveal devitalized slough or eschar within the wound bed from a lack of or inappropriate treatment. External hemorrhage is common with acute wounds and is categorized as capillary, venous, or arterial.[7] Capillary bleeding produces oozing, bright red blood. Venous bleeding presents as a steady flow of dark red blood. Arterial bleeding produces bright red blood in a squirting flow. The production of exudate is generally related to the depth of tissue damage, with deeper wounds presenting with higher levels of exudate than superficial wounds. Reassessments of exudate levels can be influenced by dressing type and, in rare cases, infection. Erythema, **maceration, denuded** tissue, **ecchymosis,** or swelling of the periwound or adjacent tissue can indicate infection, adverse reactions, or trauma to secondary structures. For example, a delayed inspection of a heavily draining wound covered with a low-absorptive dressing can reveal maceration of the periwound tissue.

Table 1-1. Wound Bed Tissue and Color[13,14]

Tissue Type	Color	Description
Granulation (see Figure 1-9)	Red, pink	Granular surface, moist, **viable**, healthy
Slough, necrotic (see Figure 1-10)	White, yellow, tan, brown, green	**Devitalized**, soft, moist, stringy or fibrous texture, loose or adhered to wound bed
Eschar, necrotic (see Figure 1-11)	Black, brown	Devitalized, **desiccated**, thick, hard or soft, loose or adhered to wound bed or perimeter
Bone, tendon, ligament (see Figure 1-12)	White/gray (bone), white/yellow (tendon and ligament)	Viable, exposed, possible damage from trauma

Color represents predominant color of the wound bed. Wounds may be multiple colors.

Figure 1-9. Granulation tissue within the wound bed.

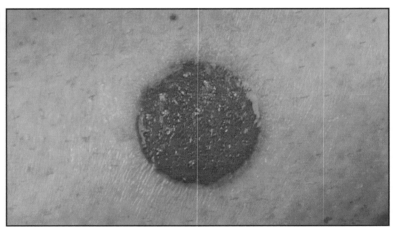

Figure 1-10. Slough within the wound bed. (Reproduced with permission from Irion G. *Comprehensive Wound Management*. 2nd ed. SLACK Inc.)

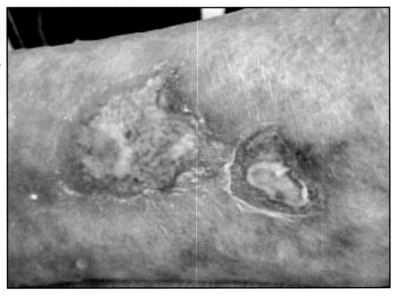

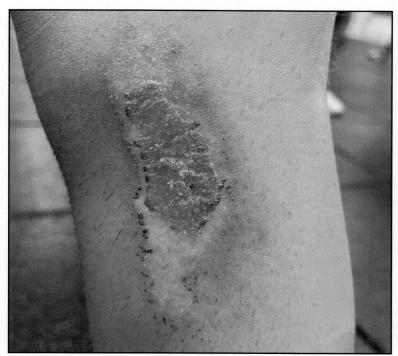

Figure 1-11. Eschar within the wound bed.

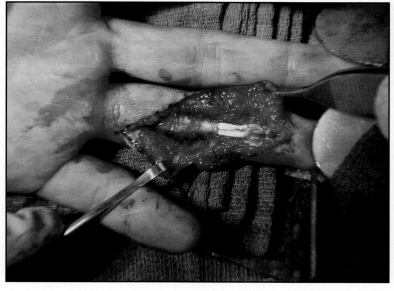

Figure 1-12. Tendon exposed within the wound bed. Note the white structure.

Excessive erythema can indicate infection or allergic contact dermatitis from a dressing. Debris (eg, dirt, sand, or foreign bodies) in the wound bed can promote the development of infection.

Palpation of soft tissues for swelling, location of pain, temperature, and deformity can indicate an associated injury or condition. Palpation is performed bilaterally, beginning away from the injured site and finishing at the periwound tissue and wound. Avoid direct contact with the wound surface and bed to prevent possible contamination and further trauma to the tissues. Swelling is detected by a change in tissue density and can identify trauma to adjacent tissues or an underlying injury.[9] Painful areas palpated away from the wound should be compared bilaterally and may indicate an associated injury. Assessment of periwound tissue temperature is performed by lightly touching the area with the dorsal surface of the hand and comparing it to the surrounding tissue to determine relative differences. Elevated skin temperatures occur immediately after activity and may also be associated with inflammation or infection. However, a decrease in temperature may signal vascular pathology. A deformity in bony alignment, joint contour, or soft tissue deficit requires further assessment and possible referral.

Range of motion and functional testing can indicate the readiness level of the patient to return to activity or work and guide treatment interventions. Bilateral active range of motion of the joints adjacent, distal, and proximal to the wound is first conducted when no associated injury or condition is suspected. With normal results, resistive range of motion and functional testing are performed to determine a return to activity. The inability of the patient to move the joint through a normal range of motion warrants further assessment for possible associated trauma. Findings from the testing may also impact dressing selection and application. For example, a patient with a partial-thickness fingertip laceration will require a low-profile, durable dressing to allow full range of motion at the distal interphalangeal joint to enter data successfully on a computer keyboard. Conversely, a patient with a full-thickness anterior knee abrasion may experience a reduction in knee flexion with dressing application, requiring a restriction in return to full activity.

Neurologic and vascular screenings are performed with deep wounds involving subcutaneous tissue, bone, or tendon or nerve injury. The neurologic screen includes sensory, motor, and reflex testing to identify nerve impingement, entrapment, or damage.[9] Vascular screening is conducted through the assessment of lower and upper extremity pulses distal to the wound and capillary refill to determine the arterial blood supply.[9]

A review of systems is included as part of a complete assessment process. Evaluation of cardiopulmonary, respiratory, gastrointestinal, and genitourinary systems is necessary for patients with deep wounds, comorbidities, a history of delayed wound healing or complications, or clinical features of infection or adverse reactions. The review can identify factors that may affect wound healing; conditions that warrant referral for further evaluation and treatment; and cleansing, debridement, and dressing interventions. Patients who return to athletic or work activities after assessment and treatment interventions may not require a system review initially. Clinicians can review the systems during reassessments as warranted.

CLINICAL DECISION-MAKING

Upon completion of the initial assessment, a clinical diagnosis and management plan are determined based on the findings and individual patient. Findings will first determine if emergent treatment and immediate referral are required. In some situations, a return-to-play decision will be needed. The clinical diagnosis is based on patient signs and symptoms and wound characteristics revealed in the primary and secondary surveys. The wound type is categorized by the depth and extent of tissue involvement, tissue color, amount and type of hemorrhage, and associated trauma. Wound categorization and assessment findings, such as a patient history of delayed healing or complications, patient occupation or activity level, wound contamination and setting, and trauma to other structures, guide the development of the management plan.

The management plan should include the types of interventions, frequency of reassessments, patient education, prediction of time required for healing and return to activity, and outcome goals. The type of wound determines the appropriate cleansing, debridement, and dressing interventions needed to create an optimal environment for healing. For example, an open, partial-thickness blister on a bony prominence may benefit from a thicker **primary** or **secondary dressing** to lessen friction forces and minimize further trauma to promote healing. A patient with a full-thickness incision over an area of high skin tension without adequate tissue approximation requires emergent treatment and referral. Reassessments should be conducted daily. The structured schedule in the athletic setting normally allows for daily assessments in the athletic training facility. Education for patients on the clinical features of infection and adverse reactions and guidelines for dressing wear can increase adherence to daily monitoring and prevent unnecessary dressing changes.[1] Most acute wounds will follow a predictable sequence of repair and achieve complete healing within weeks.[2,3] A safe return to activity or work is allowed with a low risk of reinjury, full functional ability, and achieved objectives of the intervention techniques. The goal of the management plan is to create a moist, clean, and warm wound environment to facilitate complete healing in the shortest amount of time.[1,15,16]

INITIAL MANAGEMENT

Appropriate management of acute skin trauma involves prompt recognition and assessment of the patient with immediate and follow-up interventions to promote healing and lessen the risk of adverse reactions. After the primary and secondary surveys, immediate management of wounds in the athletic setting is commonly performed on the field or court or in an athletic training facility. This initial cleansing, debridement, and dressing of the wound to allow the patient a timely return to activity must be followed after activity with a more comprehensive assessment in the athletic training facility.[1] Daily monitoring and reassessments of the patient, wound bed, periwound tissue, and dressing should be conducted to determine the effectiveness of the interventions, identify possible development of adverse reactions, and guide dressing changes and revisions to the management plan.

In some situations, referral of the patient with acute skin trauma or activation of the emergency action plan is necessary. Organizations and institutions should develop and implement a written emergency action plan that defines the personnel, equipment, communication system, emergency transportation, location (eg, soccer practice field or aquatic center), emergency medical facilities, and documentation procedures.[17] If a referral is necessary after the assessment, thorough cleansing, debridement, and dressing of the wound are not required. In these cases, promptly cover the wound with sterile gauze, apply a secondary dressing, and refer. Immobilization of the body part should be considered to prevent movement and lessen further trauma. Acute skin trauma injuries that require referral are listed in Table 1-2.

SUMMARY

Acute skin trauma results from external shear and tensile forces and tensile loads and results in various injuries to the skin. Assessment of skin trauma consists of primary and secondary surveys to identify a clinical diagnosis, patient factors that may affect healing, and treatment interventions. Clinicians perform the primary survey to identify emergent injuries and conditions. The clinician assesses patient and wound history, inspects and palpates the involved and adjacent body areas, evaluates readiness levels for activity, and reviews systems for associated trauma and conditions with the secondary survey. The clinical presentation of acute wounds is based on the severity of trauma and the resultant tissue damage. The clinician integrates the assessment findings to determine a clinical diagnosis and develop a management plan for the patient and wound.

Table 1-2. Acute Skin Trauma Requiring Referral[1,7]

Clinical features involving the following:

- Uncontrolled external hemorrhage
- Moderate loss of soft tissue
- Heavy, visible contamination
- Wounds associated with a fracture
- Animal or human bite
- Unsuccessful **tissue approximation**
- Unremovable embedded objects
- Lapse of tetanus immunization
- Deep wounds compromising subcutaneous tissue, tendon, or nerve
- Wounds that receive delayed treatment
- Patients with **immunocompromised** conditions
- Presence of numbness or tingling
- Wound infection: Fever, pain, edema, erythema, warmth, wound **dehiscence**, and delayed wound healing
- Adverse reactions: **Erythematous** rash, **eczematous** reaction, **vesicles**, white discoloration, tenderness, nodularity, burning, **pruritus**, or systemic reactions, including **urticarial** and **anaphylaxis**

REFERENCES

1. Beam JW, Buckley B, Holcomb W, Ciocca M. National Athletic Trainers' Association position statement: Management of acute skin trauma. *J Athl Train.* 2016;51(12):1053-1070.

2. Lazarus GS, Cooper DM, Knighton DR, et al. Definitions and guidelines for assessment of wounds and evaluation of healing. *Arch Dermatol.* 1994;130(4):489-493.

3. Lee CK, Hansen SL. Management of acute wounds. *Surg Clin North Am.* 2009;89(3):659-676.

4. Honsik KA, Romeo MW, Hawley CJ, Romeo SJ, Romeo JP. Sideline skin and wound care for acute injuries. *Curr Sports Med Rep.* 2007;6(3):147-154.

5. Hussey M, Bagg M. Principles of wound closure. *Oper Tech Sports Med.* 2011;19:206-211.

6. Davidson JM. Animal models for wound repair. *Arch Dermatol Res.* 1998;290(suppl):S1-S11.

7. Miller MG, Berry DC. Recognition and management of soft tissue injuries. In: Miller MG, Berry DC, eds. *Emergency Response Management for Athletic Trainers.* Wolters Kluwer/Lippincott Williams and Wilkins; 2010:283-309.

8. Beam JW, Beck F. Soft-tissue injury management. In: Starkey C, ed. *Athletic Training and Sports Medicine: An Integrated Approach.* 5th ed. Jones & Barlett Learning; 2012:13-36.

9. Starkey C, Ryan SD. *Examination of Orthopedic & Athletic Injuries.* 4th ed. F.A. Davis; 2015.

10. Franz MG, Steed DL, Robson MC. Optimizing healing of the acute wound by minimizing complications. *Curr Probl Surg.* 2007;44(11):691-763.

11. Hess CT, Kirsner RS. Orchestrating wound healing: Assessing and preparing the wound bed. *Adv Skin Wound Care.* 2003;16(5):246-257.

12. Nicks BA, Ayello EA, Woo K, Nitzki-George D, Sibbald RG. Acute wound management: Revisiting the approach to assessment, irrigation, and closure considerations. *Int J Emerg Med.* 2010;3(4):399-407.

13. Brown G. Wound documentation: Managing risk. *Adv Skin Wound Care.* 2006;19(3):155-165, quiz 165-167.

14. Lampe, KE. The general evaluation. In: McCulloch, JM, Kloth, LC, eds. *Wound Healing: Evidence-Based Management.* 4th ed. F.A. Davis; 2010:65-93.

15. Thomas S. A structured approach to the selection of dressings. World Wide Wounds. 1997. Accessed June 25, 2021. http://www.worldwidewounds.com/1997/july/Thomas-Guide/Dress-Select.html

16. Beam JW. Effects of occlusive dressings on healing of partial-thickness abrasions. *Athl Train Sports Health Care.* 2012;4(2):58-66.

17. Anderson JC, Courson RW, Kleiner DM. National Athletic Trainers' Association position statement: Emergency planning in athletics. *J Athl Train.* 2002;37(1):99-104.

2

INFECTION CONTROL AND STANDARD PRECAUTIONS

In the appropriate management of acute skin trauma, clinicians must adhere to the facility and organizational guidelines, standards, and procedures to lessen the risk of adverse events. The overall goals of preventative measures are to reduce the risk of infection and adverse reactions, protect personnel from potentially infectious agents, and maintain a clean environment and facility. This chapter focuses on infection control guidelines and procedures and includes standard precautions, hand hygiene, personal protective equipment (PPE), and cleaning and disinfection. Sterile and clean techniques and facility and environmental considerations are presented next. This is followed by a discussion on procedures to minimize the transmission of microorganisms among patients, clinicians and personnel, equipment, and the environment during assessment and cleansing, debridement, and dressing interventions. The chapter concludes with recommended wound management supplies for athletic training facilities and medical kits.

INFECTION CONTROL

Infection control procedures are critical in preventing infection and adverse reactions in managing acute skin trauma. All personnel and facilities involved in wound care should develop

DOI: 10.1201/9781003523055-2

policies and procedures that address preventative measures and enforce adherence to the practices to reduce the risk of adverse outcomes. Infection control measures include standard precautions, hand hygiene, PPE, and facility and equipment cleaning and disinfection.

Standard Precautions

Standard precautions extend universal precautions and should be followed during the management of acute skin trauma. According to **universal precautions**, all blood and body fluid are treated as if known to be **infectious**.[1] **Standard precautions** view all patients as potentially infected or colonized with organisms capable of being transmitted.[2] Standard precautions provide the minimum infection control procedures for patient health care and involve hand hygiene and PPE.

Hand Hygiene

Hand hygiene is considered the single most important practice to lessen the transmission of infectious agents.[3-5] Clinicians should perform handwashing when the hands are visibly dirty or soiled[3]; before contact with a patient[6,7]; if moving from a **contaminated** wound to a clean wound on a patient[2]; after contact with a patient's skin[7-10]; after contact with blood, body fluid, nonintact skin, or wound dressings[6]; after contact with **inanimate** surfaces and objects (medical equipment)[11-16]; and after the removal of gloves.[17-19] Hands are washed with either nonantimicrobial soap and water or antimicrobial soap and water when visibly dirty or contaminated[3] or **decontaminated** with an alcohol-based hand rub when not visibly dirty.[20,21] To wash the hands, wet the hands with water, apply the recommended amount of soap to the hands, rub the hands together vigorously for at least 15 seconds, rinse the hands with water, and dry thoroughly with a disposable towel.[3] To decontaminate the hands, apply an alcohol-based hand rub onto the palm of a hand and rub the hands and fingers together until the surfaces are dry.[22,23]

Personal Protective Equipment

PPE is a barrier to protect the clinician from infectious agents.[2] PPE should be worn when an anticipated patient interaction may involve contact with blood or body fluid.[2] Appropriate PPE does not allow infectious materials to pass through or reach the clinician's clothes, skin, eyes, mouth, or other mucous membranes under normal conditions.[1] PPE for acute wound management includes gloves, a mask, goggles or glasses, a face shield, and protective clothing.

Gloves protect the patient and clinician from infectious agents carried on the hands.[12] A single pair of clean, boxed examination gloves provide adequate barrier protection for contact with blood and body fluid.[24] Sterile gloves are required for procedures performed in a sterile field, such as wound closure with sutures or staples. The glove material used is based on facility availability and clinician preference. However, latex or nitrile gloves may be preferable for techniques that require manual dexterity.[2] Gloves should be changed between patients, after contact with the surrounding environment or equipment, during interventions on a single patient if treating a contaminated body area and moving to a clean area, and if torn or punctured.[1,2] Gloves should not be reused and should be disposed of in a designated area or container per facility policies and procedures. Handwashing should be performed before applying gloves (Tables 2-1 and 2-2) and after removal (Table 2-3).

Table 2-1. Application of Examination Gloves

Remove a glove from the box. Touch only the cuff at the top edge of the glove (Figure 2-1).	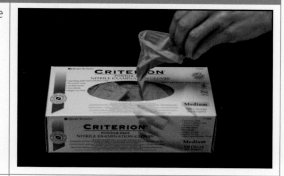 **Figure 2-1**
Insert the fingers and thumb (Figure 2-2) and apply the first glove (Figure 2-3).	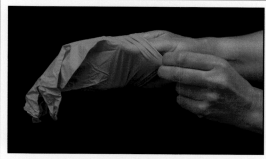 **Figure 2-2** 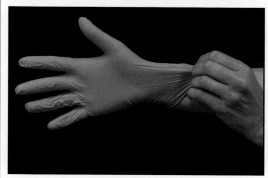 **Figure 2-3**
Remove the second glove from the box with the bare hand and touch only the cuff at the top edge (Figure 2-4).	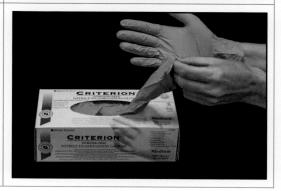 **Figure 2-4**

continued

Table 2-1. Application of Examination Gloves (continued)

Avoid touching the skin of the forearm with the gloved hand. Fold the cuff over the fingers of the gloved hand, insert the fingers and thumb, and apply the second glove (Figure 2-5). **Figure 2-5**	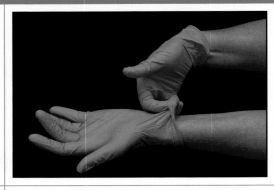
Once gloved, proceed to the procedure requiring gloves.	
Gloves are applied after other personal protective equipment. If a gown is worn, gloves should cover the gown wrist cuffs.	

Table 2-2. Application of Sterile Gloves

Open the outer packaging to expose the inner wrapping containing the sterile gloves (Figure 2-6).	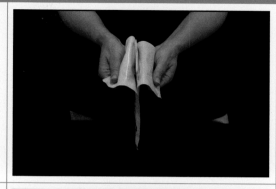**Figure 2-6**
Hold the outer packaging and place the inner wrapping and gloves on a clean, dry table (Figure 2-7).	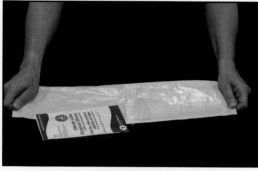**Figure 2-7**
Pinch the outer edges and unfold the inner wrapping (Figure 2-8).	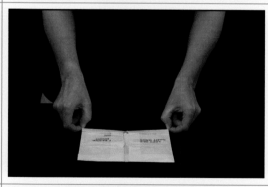**Figure 2-8**
Unfold the bottom (Figure 2-9) and then the top (Figure 2-10) corners of the inner packaging by the corners.	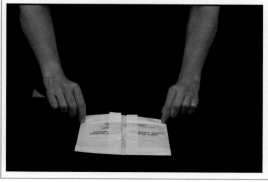**Figure 2-9**

continued

Table 2-2. Application of Sterile Gloves (continued)

Figure 2-10	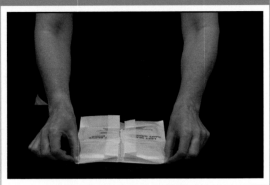
Completely unfold the packaging sleeves (Figure 2-11). Avoid touching the packaging where the gloves make contact. **Figure 2-11**	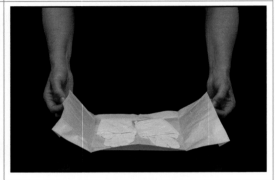
Pick up the first glove on the folded cuff with the thumb and first finger of the bare hand (Figure 2-12). **Figure 2-12**	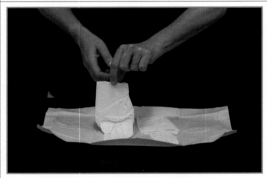
Insert the fingers and thumb and pull the glove with the bare hand on the folded cuff (Figure 2-13). **Figure 2-13**	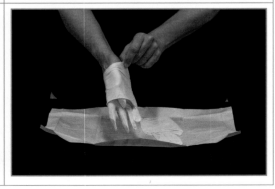

continued

Table 2-2. Application of Sterile Gloves (continued)

Pinch the palmar aspect of the folded cuff with the bare fingers and pull until the cuff is extended onto the wrist (Figure 2-14).	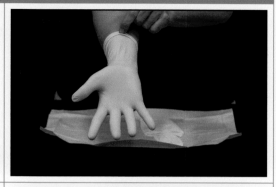 **Figure 2-14**
Place the fingers (eg, second and third) of the gloved hand inside the folded cuff of the second glove (Figure 2-15).	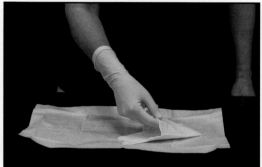 **Figure 2-15**
Insert the fingers and thumb and apply the second glove using the gloved fingers for assistance (Figure 2-16).	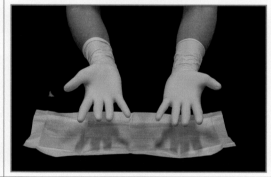 **Figure 2-16**
Once gloved, proceed to the procedure requiring gloves.	
Gloves are applied after other personal protective equipment. If a gown is worn, gloves should cover the gown wrist cuffs.	

Table 2-3. Removal of Gloves

Grasp one glove at the palm/cuff area (Figure 2-17) and peel the first glove off, turning it inside out.	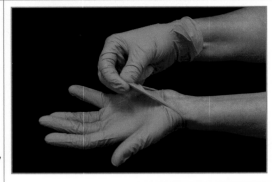 **Figure 2-17**
Avoid touching the skin of the forearm with the gloved hand.	
Keep the removed glove in the gloved hand (Figure 2-18).	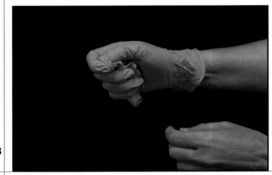 **Figure 2-18**
Insert the finger(s) of the ungloved hand under the cuff of the second glove (Figure 2-19) and peel off, turning it inside out over the first glove (Figure 2-20).	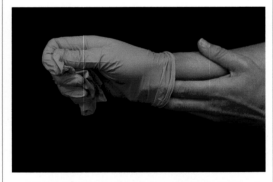 **Figure 2-19** 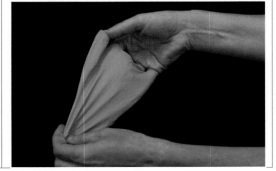 **Figure 2-20**

continued

Table 2-3. Removal of Gloves (continued)	
Dispose of gloves as directed by facility policies and procedures.	
Gloves are the first personal protective equipment removed.	

Masks, goggles, glasses, and face shields should be worn with procedures that produce a splash, spatter, or spray of blood or body fluid to protect the eyes, nose, and mouth from contamination.[1] **Splash back** can occur during irrigation of the wound bed and should be anticipated. Masks covering the nose and mouth can be used with goggles or glasses with lateral shields to lessen mouth, nose, and eye exposure. Alternatively, a mask worn with a disposable or nondisposable, chin-length face shield provides enhanced protection to the eyes and other facial areas not covered with goggles or glasses. Personal glasses and contact lenses worn alone do not adequately protect the eyes.[2] The use of glasses or contact lenses during techniques will require goggles or a face shield for protection.

Protective clothing such as gowns, aprons, or lab coats protects exposed body areas (eg, arms) and clothing from contamination with infectious agents. The protective clothing should extend from the neck to midthigh or below and fully cover the arms and anterior body.[2] Coats worn in routine clinical settings are not appropriate for use as protective clothing.

The application and removal of PPE follow a standard sequence to lessen the risk of contaminating clothing, skin, and mucous membranes with infectious materials.[2] The application of PPE begins with handwashing. Next, protective clothing is applied followed by a mask. Goggles, glasses, or a face shield are placed over the face and eyes. Lastly, gloves are applied and should cover the wrist or cuff of the protective clothing. During the removal of PPE, clinicians must remember that the outside or front surfaces of PPE are contaminated and should not be touched. Additionally, handwashing should occur immediately before proceeding if the hands become contaminated with the removal of any PPE during the sequence. First, remove gloves and perform handwashing. Remove the goggles or glasses from the earpieces or face shield by the headband from the head and face. Next, remove the protective clothing by pulling it away from the torso, touching only the inside surface, and then turning it inside out into a bundle. Lastly, grasp the ties or bands of the mask and remove them. Clinicians can also perform PPE removal by removing the protective clothing and gloves together and then the goggles, glasses, or face shields and the mask. Perform handwashing when PPE removal is complete.

Cleaning and Disinfection

Cleaning and **disinfection** procedures are essential in preventing and controlling infectious agents. Standard precautions and cleaning and disinfection practices must become an organizational norm for all personnel.[25] Organizations should develop and implement a written schedule for cleaning and disinfection and decontamination methods based on the venue location, type of surface, type of soil (eg, blood), and wound management techniques.[1] Follow hand hygiene and PPE procedures during cleaning and disinfection.

Cleaning and disinfection of environmental surfaces (eg, tabletops, cabinet tops, and floors) should occur on a regular basis and when visibly soiled; likely to be contaminated; after contact with blood or body fluid; and after completion of cleansing, debridement, or dressing procedures.[1,2] Surfaces that are frequently touched (eg, treatment tables and cabinets) should receive more frequent cleaning and disinfection.[2] Spills of blood or other potentially infectious agents should be cleaned and disinfected immediately.[1] Large amounts of fluid can first be cleaned with disposable, absorbent cloth or paper towels. Select the cleaning solutions, such as soap or detergent, and follow the manufacturers' recommendations on use. Select disinfection solutions registered by the Environmental Protection Agency and follow the manufacturers' instructions for the amount, dilution, safe use, contact time, storage, shelf life, and disposal.[2,26]

Instruments should undergo a cleaning, disinfection, and **sterilization** process based on the level of contact with tissue. Instruments that enter or contact viable tissue, such as tweezers or forceps used to pack a puncture wound, should be cleaned with water and detergent immediately after use and then high-level disinfected or sterilized.[26] Instruments that do not contact viable tissue (eg, scissors) are cleaned and disinfected with a registered Environmental Protection Agency solution after each use, when visibly soiled, and on a regular basis.[26] Sterile, disposable tweezers, forceps, and scissors are an option for the clinician.

Contaminated laundry (eg, towels and reusable protective clothing) should be collected in separate bags or containers immediately after use. Handle the laundry with a minimum of agitation to avoid further contamination and monitor the bag or container for leakage of fluids.[1] A hot or cold water cycle is used for washing. Follow the manufacturers' recommendations for the type, concentration, and amount of detergent, cycle time, and fabric care instructions.[1]

Medical waste should be contained and disposed of in the wound treatment area.[1,27] Place items contaminated with blood or wound drainage (eg, gauze, dressings, and cleaning and disinfection supplies) in a biohazard container. Place sharp instruments (eg, disposable tweezers, forceps, and scissors) in appropriate sharps containers.[1,27] Organizations must have a plan for collecting, handling, and disposing of medical waste in their policy and procedure manual.

STERILE AND CLEAN TECHNIQUES

Two approaches are used in the management of acute skin trauma: sterile and clean techniques. Sterile is the absence of microorganisms in the environment. This environment is found in operating or surgical suites. The **sterile technique** uses procedures to reduce exposure to microorganisms and maintain the environment as free from microorganisms as possible.[28] This technique includes handwashing; creating and maintaining a sterile field; and the use of sterile PPE, instruments, and supplies (eg, dressings, towels, and linens) for cleansing, debridement, and dressing of the wound. A sterile-to-sterile procedure is used, meaning only sterile material should contact the wound.[29] Clean is an environment free of dirt or gross contamination. The **clean technique** is the use of procedures to reduce the overall number of microorganisms or reduce the risk of transmission of microorganisms among clinicians, patients, and locations.[28] This technique involves handwashing; creating and maintaining a clean field; and the use of sterile instruments and clean PPE and supplies. The clean technique allows for the use of clean, boxed examination gloves and clean towels and linens in a clean vs sterile environment. Sterile-to-sterile procedures are not used with a clean technique.[28] See Table 2-4 for sterile and clean technique supplies and equipment.

Clinical decisions regarding the appropriate use of sterile or clean techniques to lessen the risk of infection, adverse reactions, and contamination can be confusing for clinicians. The available research and literature provide no clear evidence for differences in the rates of infection and healing of acute and chronic wounds with the use of the sterile or clean technique. Additionally, expert opinion differs on standard definitions of the sterile and clean technique and when each technique is warranted. A limited number of guidelines and recommendations have been published on the use of sterile and clean techniques for the management of acute wounds. The Centers for Disease Control and Prevention[30] recommend the sterile technique for 24 to 48 hours in the management of postoperative incisions. Further recommendations beyond this period are not provided. The Wound, Ostomy, and Continence Nurses Society[28] noted sterile techniques for patients with an increased risk of infection, for invasive procedures (eg, sharp instrumental debridement), and in acute hospital settings for the management of chronic wounds. The clean technique is suggested for

Table 2-4. Sterile and Clean Technique Supplies and Equipment
Sterile
• Sterile gloves • Sterile personal protective equipment • Sterile instruments (eg, forceps, tweezers, and scissors), equipment, and supplies • Unopened solutions, dressings, and ointments
Clean
• Sterile instruments (eg, forceps and tweezers) • Clean scissors • Clean, boxed examination gloves • Clean personal protective equipment • Clean equipment and supplies

patients not at a high risk of infection, routine dressing changes, and wounds healing by secondary intention through the formation of granulation tissue.[28] Clinicians should consider patient, wound, procedure, setting, and material factors in the selection of the sterile or clean technique. Patient comorbidities such as diabetes and immunocompromise, wounds that expose deep tissues and structures or receive delayed treatment, invasive procedures such as packing a full-thickness puncture wound, wound management in unknown or contaminated locations or venues, and the availability and use of sterile and clean supplies and equipment can increase the risk of contamination and infection. The creation of an actual sterile environment found in a surgical suite is not possible in an athletic training facility. However, clinicians can create a clean environment and use sterile PPE, instruments, and supplies to prevent contamination and infection. Referrals of patients for advanced cleansing, debridement, and dressing techniques that require a sterile environment and technique should be performed. Physician examination rooms or appropriate spaces in the treatment area of an athletic training facility can be created and maintained as a clean environment. Clinicians should develop policies and procedures addressing the use of sterile and clean techniques following published recommendations. Next, cleansing, debridement, and dressing procedures and techniques are discussed to lessen the risk of contamination during the management of the patient and wound.

PROCEDURES AND TECHNIQUES

Wound management procedures and techniques must be performed with infection control guidelines to lessen the risk of transmission of infectious agents. Clinicians should prepare the treatment area, and all supplies and equipment should be gathered and brought to the area before the procedure. When using the clean technique, clean and disinfect and then cover tabletops with clean towels or linens. Towels are needed with irrigation to absorb and control excess cleansing solutions to lessen the risk of contamination of tables and floors. All supplies and equipment should remain unopened in the original packaging until ready to use. If additional supplies are needed during a procedure, have other personnel gather and open the items. If the clinician needs to gather additional items, remove gloves, obtain the supplies, perform handwashing, and apply new gloves.[29] The remaining supplies used with the clean technique that can be used again should be stored in their original packaging and used on the same patient.[29] Packages and containers of topical antibiotics or ointments should be restricted for use on a single patient. Multiple wounds on a single patient are managed individually. Wounds with clinical features of infection or adverse reactions should be treated last if the patient presents with multiple wounds.[31] Following the completion of these procedures, clinicians must adhere to facility infection control practices for cleaning and disinfection of contaminated treatment area surfaces, instruments, and laundry and proper disposal of waste.

Several techniques for cleansing, debridement, and dressing procedures can reduce the risk of contamination, infection, and transmission of microorganisms. When using the clean technique with noninfected wounds, a cupped hand, splash guard, or cup with a hole lessen splash back from irrigation for the clinician and patient (see Chapter 3). The **no-touch technique** can reduce the risk of contamination during dressing application and changes. Clinicians should cut (if necessary), handle, and apply the dressing by touching only the border(s), avoiding touching any portion of the dressing that will contact the wound bed.[28,29] Dressings should remain in place over the wound bed until dressing changes are necessary to lessen contamination of the wound. Dressing changes are based on the recommended wear times and wound status or the development of dressing integrity issues, clinical infection, or adverse reactions.

WOUND MANAGEMENT SUPPLIES

Athletic training facilities and medical kits should have supplies and equipment for the management of acute skin trauma readily available. The facility will be used for comprehensive management techniques and contain a selection of cleansing solutions and equipment, debridement supplies, nonocclusive and occlusive dressings, and infection control supplies (Table 2-5). Clinicians should store these supplies and equipment at room temperature in a dry area. Wound cleansing and debridement solutions, dressings, and environmental cleaners and disinfectants have expiration dates. Inventory regularly and rotate these supplies as needed. A similar selection of supplies and equipment can be packed into trunks or bags for team travel.

Athletic training medical kits require minimal supplies during practices and competitions (Table 2-6). As discussed in Chapter 5, nonocclusive dressings are best suited for covering wounds during practices and competitions with follow-up cleansing, debridement, and dressing techniques performed in the facility. Clinicians should shield kits from direct sunlight and excessive heat, humidity, and moisture to prevent damage to solutions and dressings. Clinicians can use small closable plastic bags or containers to store supplies in kits for further protection.

SUMMARY

Facilities and clinicians should develop and adhere to prevention measures to reduce the risk of infection and adverse outcomes. Infection control procedures and standard precautions guide acute wound management techniques among all patients and settings. The appropriate use of handwashing and PPE consisting of gloves, masks, goggles or glasses, face shields, and protective clothing can lessen the risk of transmission and protect the patient and clinician from infection. Policies and procedures should establish the cleaning and disinfection of environmental surfaces and wound care supplies and equipment. Cleansing, debridement, and dressing procedures are performed with the sterile or clean technique. The clean technique is appropriate for most patients with acute skin trauma. Athletic training facilities and medical kits should contain supplies and equipment to manage acute wounds using infection control practices.

Table 2-5. Athletic Training Facility Supplies and Equipment

Solutions and Ointments

- Normal saline
- Potable tap water
- Topical antiseptics
- Tincture of benzoin
- Topical antibiotics

Dressings

- Woven and nonwoven sterile gauze
- Impregnated sterile gauze
- Nonadherent pads
- Adhesive strips and patches
- Wound closure strips
- Alginates
- Films
- Foams
- Hydrogels
- Hydrocolloids
- Dermal adhesives
- Adhesive gauze (Cover-Roll [BSN Medical] or Omnifix [Hartmann USA])
- Nonadherent, self-adherent, or adherent tapes and wraps
- Skin tape
- Pre-wrap

Instruments

- Sterile forceps, tweezers, and scissors (disposable or reusable)
- Clean scissors

Equipment

- 35-mL syringe
- 18- to 20-gauge needle hub or plastic cannula
- Clean basins and cups
- Surgical scrub brush
- High-porosity sponge
- Clean towels or linens

Infection Control

- Antimicrobial and nonantimicrobial soap
- Alcohol-based hand rub
- Clean, boxed examination gloves
- Sterile gloves
- Masks
- Goggles or glasses

continued

Table 2-5. Athletic Training Facility Supplies and Equipment (continued)

- Face shields
- Gown, apron, or lab coat
- Biohazard container
- Sharps container
- Cleaning solutions (eg, soap or detergent)
- Disinfectants (Environmental Protection Agency registered, https://www.epa.gov/pesticide-registration/selected-epa-registered-disinfectants)

Wound Closure[a]

- Suture kit or sterile needle holder, forceps, and scissors
- Variety of suture material
- Suture removal kit or sterile suture scissors and tweezers or forceps
- Skin stapler
- Staple remover tool

[a]Based on state laws and practice acts.

Table 2-6. Athletic Training Medical Kit Supplies and Equipment

Solutions

- Normal saline
- Potable tap water
- Topical antiseptics

Dressings

- Woven and nonwoven sterile gauze
- Nonadherent pads
- Adhesive strips and patches
- Adhesive gauze (Cover-Roll [BSN Medical] or Omnifix [Hartmann USA])
- Nonadherent, self-adherent, or adherent tapes and wraps
- Skin tape
- Pre-wrap

Instruments

- Clean scissors

Equipment

- 35-mL syringe
- 18- to 20-gauge needle hub or plastic cannula
- Clean basins and cups
- Clean towels or linens

Infection Control

- Antimicrobial and nonantimicrobial soap
- Alcohol-based hand rub
- Clean, boxed examination gloves
- Masks
- Goggles or glasses
- Face shields
- Gown, apron, or lab coat
- Biohazard container
- Cleaning solutions (eg, soap or detergent)
- Disinfectants (Environmental Protection Agency registered, https://www.epa.gov/pesticide-registration/selected-epa-registered-disinfectants)

REFERENCES

1. US Department of Labor Occupational Safety & Health Administration. *Bloodborne pathogens standard.* May 2019. Accessed December 16, 2021. https://www.osha.gov/laws-regs/regulations/standardnumber/1910/1910.1030

2. Centers for Disease Control and Prevention. *2007 guideline for isolation precautions: Preventing transmission of infectious agents in healthcare settings.* July 2019. Accessed December 16, 2012. https://www.cdc.gov/infectioncontrol/pdf/guidelines/isolation-guidelines-H.pdf

3. Centers for Disease Control and Prevention. Guideline for hand hygiene in health-care settings: Recommendations of the Healthcare Infection Control Practices Advisory Committee and the HICPAC/SHEA/APIC/IDSA Hand Hygiene Task Force. *MMWR Morb Mortal Wkly Rep.* 2002;51(RR-16):1-45.

4. Jarvis WR. Handwashing—The Semmelweis lesson forgotten? *Lancet.* 1994;344(8933):1311-1312.

5. Daniels IR, Rees BI. Handwashing: Simple, but effective. *Ann R Coll Surg Engl.* 1999;81:117.

6. Semmelweiss IP. *Die Aetiologie, der Begriff und Die Prophylaxis des Kindbettfiebers.* C.A. Harleben's Verlags-Expedition; 1861.

7. Mortimer EA Jr, Lipsitz PJ, Wolinsky E, Gonzaga AJ, Rammelkamp CH Jr. Transmission of *Staphylococci* between newborns. Importance of the hands to personnel. *Am J Dis Child.* 1962;104:289-295.

8. McFarland LV, Mulligan ME, Kwok RY, Stamm WE. Nosocomial acquisition of *Clostridium difficile* infection. *N Engl J Med.* 1989;320(4):204-210.

9. Ehrenkranz NJ, Alfonso BC. Failure of bland soap handwash to prevent hand transfer of patient bacteria to urethral catheters. *Infect Control Hosp Epidemiol.* 1991;12(11):654-662.

10. Casewell M, Phillips I. Hands as route of transmission for *Klebsiella* species. *Br Med J.* 1977;2(6098):1315-1317.

11. Bhalla A, Pultz NJ, Gries DM, et al. Acquisition of nosocomial pathogens on hands after contact with environmental surfaces near hospitalized patients. *Infect Control Hosp Epidemiol.* 2004;25(2):164-167.

12. Duckro AN, Blom DW, Lyle EA, Weinstein RA, Hayden MK. Transfer of vancomycin-resistant *enterococci* via health care worker hands. *Arch Intern Med.* 2005;165(3):302-307.

13. Boyce JM, Potter-Bynoe G, Chenevert C, King T. Environmental contamination due to methicillin-resistant *Staphylococcus aureus:* Possible infection control implications. *Infect Control Hosp Epidemiol.* 1997;18(9):622-627.

14. Samore MH, Venkataraman L, DeGirolami PC, Arbeit RD, Karchmer AW. Clinical and molecular epidemiology of sporadic and clustered cases of nosocomial *Clostridium difficile* diarrhea. *Am J Med.* 1996;100(1):32-40.

15. Ojajarvi J. Effectiveness of hand washing and disinfection methods in removing transient bacteria after patient nursing. *J Hyg (Lond).* 1980;85(2):193-203.

16. Otter J, Havill N, Adams N, Joyce J. *Extensive environmental contamination associated with patients with loose stools and MRSA colonization of the gastrointestinal tract.* Paper presented at: 16th Annual Scientific Meeting of the Society for Healthcare Epidemiology of America; March 18-21, 2006; Chicago, IL. Abstract 159.

17. Tenorio AR, Badri SM, Sahgal NB, et al. Effectiveness of gloves in the prevention of hand carriage of vancomycin-resistant *enterococcus* species by health care workers after patient care. *Clin Infect Dis.* 2001;32(5):826-829.

18. Olsen RJ, Lynch P, Coyle MB, Cummings J, Bokete T, Stamm WE. Examination gloves as barriers to hand contamination in clinical practice. *JAMA.* 1993;270(3):350-353.

19. Doebbeling BN, Pfaller MA, Houston AK, Wenzel RP. Removal of nosocomial pathogens from the contaminated glove. Implications for glove reuse and handwashing. *Ann Intern Med.* 1988;109(5):394-398.

20. Pittet D, Hugonnet S, Harbarth S, et al. Effectiveness of a hospital-wide programme to improve compliance with hand hygiene. Infection Control Programme. *Lancet.* 2000;356(9238):1307-1312.

21. Widmer AF. Replace hand washing with use of a waterless alcohol hand rub? *Clin Infect Dis.* 2000;31(1):136-143.

22. Taylor LJ. An evaluation of handwashing techniques-1. *Nursing Times.* 1978:54-55.

23. Ojajärvi J. An evaluation of antiseptics used for hand disinfection in wards. *J Hyg (Lond).* 1976;76:75-82.

24. Korniewicz DM, Kirwin M, Cresci K, et al. Barrier protection with examination gloves: Double versus single. *Am J Infect Control.* 1994;22(1):12-15.

25. Zinder SM, Basler RSW, Foley J, Scarlata C, Vasily DB. National Athletic Trainers' Association position statement: Skin diseases. *J Athl Train.* 2010;45(4):411-428.

26. Centers for Disease Control and Prevention. *Guideline for disinfection and sterilization in healthcare facilities, 2008.* May 2019. Accessed December 24, 2021. https://www.cdc.gov/infection-control/pdf/guidelines/disinfection-guidelines-H.pdf

27. Centers for Disease Control and Prevention. *Guidelines for environmental infection control in health-care facilities.* July 2019. Accessed December 24, 2021. https://www.cdc.gov/infection-control/pdf/guidelines/environmental-guidelines-P.pdf

28. Wound, Ostomy and Continence Nurses Society Wound Committee; Association for Professionals in Infection Control and Epidemiology, Inc, 2000 Guidelines Committee. Clean vs. sterile dressing techniques for management of chronic wounds. *J Wound Ostomy Continence Nurs.* 2012;39(2 suppl):S30-S34.

29. Myers BA. *Wound Management: Principles and Practice.* Pearson Prentice Hall; 2008:94-122.

30. Berríos-Torres SI, Umscheid CA, Bratzler DW, et al. Centers for Disease Control and Prevention guideline for the prevention of surgical site infection, 2017. *JAMA Surg.* 2017;152(8):784-791.

31. Faller NA. Clean versus sterile: A review of the literature. *Ostomy Wound Manage.* 1999;45(5):56-60, 62, 64 passim.

3

CLEANSING

Bernadette Buckley, PhD, LAT, ATC

Cleansing is often the first step in managing acute skin trauma. Cleansing involves the application of a nontoxic solution to the wound bed to facilitate the removal of exudate, microorganisms, debris, and dressing residue.[1-3] Cleansing interventions precede debridement and dressing selection and application. The similarities between cleansing and debridement often result in some clinicians viewing wound debridement as part of wound cleansing, whereas others consider it distinctly different.[4] Because of this discrepancy in the definition of cleansing and the limited high-quality evidence to guide clinical practice, clinicians often rely on personal preferences or ritualistic practices in selecting interventions. This chapter begins with a discussion of the goal and purposes of cleansing. Next, patient, wound, and clinician factors to consider in technique selection are presented. This is followed by a discussion on cleansing techniques, including indications, contraindications, and procedures, for acute wounds. The chapter concludes with cleansing solutions and the appropriate solution temperature to facilitate healing and minimize the risk of infection and adverse reactions among acute skin trauma.

DOI: 10.1201/9781003523055-3

CLEANSING GOAL AND PURPOSES

Acute skin trauma sustained in athletic, recreational, and work activities is initially considered contaminated with organic and inorganic foreign bodies.[4] Initial cleansing of acute wounds is necessary to remove nonviable debris and lessen the risk of adverse outcomes. The goal of cleansing is to create a clean, moist, and warm environment that is conducive to healing. The purposes of cleansing are to remove debris, exudate, microorganisms, and metabolic waste from the wound bed and periwound tissue.[5,6] Cleansing allows for a clear visual inspection and assessment of the tissues to determine a clinical diagnosis and develop the management plan. Clinicians can also use cleansing to rehydrate a desiccated wound to create and maintain a moist environment and minimize tissue trauma during dressing changes.[5,7-9] In addition to the physiological benefits of cleansing to remove any material that can delay healing, a psychological component should be considered.[4] Cleansing interventions provide patients with an overall sense of health and well-being during the healing process.[10-12]

FACTORS TO CONSIDER FOR CLEANSING

The selection of an appropriate cleansing technique and solution is based on several factors, including the health status and preferences of the patient, characteristics of the wound, frequency of cleansing, and clinician knowledge and experience. Clinicians should consider the patient's health status in determining the appropriate cleansing technique and solution. Sensitivity to certain chemicals found in topical **antiseptics** will exclude their use with cleansing techniques. The mechanical forces associated with scrubbing and swabbing and hydrotherapy techniques can produce pain and are inappropriate for patients with a low threshold. Patient expectations and preferences can influence technique selection, and clinicians must consider whether the benefits outweigh the risk.[4] Patients benefit from the feeling of cleanliness and often believe frequent cleansing is the proper method to treat wounds.[4] Clinicians should educate patients on the goals and rationale of interventions and explain how unnecessary dressing changes to perform frequent cleansing may delay healing and increase the risk of cross-contamination and infection.

Wound factors can influence the selection of cleansing techniques and solutions for the patient. Clinicians should consider the etiology of the wound, depth of tissue damage, presence of foreign debris, and clinical features of infection and adverse reactions. The mechanism, time, and location of the injury can reveal the depth of tissue involvement, condition of the wound bed, and level of contamination. Based on the presumed contamination following injury, all superficial- to full-thickness wounds should undergo an initial cleansing. Wounds that are deep or expose bone, muscle, tendon, nerve, or blood vessels are often covered with sterile gauze and a secondary dressing and referred for more advanced cleansing, debridement, and closure interventions. If cleansing of these wounds is considered, normal saline is the preferred solution.[13] Delayed reporting of a wound can result in the development of eschar. The patient can present with eschar covering the wound bed at the initial assessment. Debridement of the eschar will be required before thorough assessment and cleansing of the wound bed. Delayed reporting and closure of lacerations and incisions can increase the risk of infection. Clinicians may consider using topical antiseptics to cleanse the periwound tissue with these wounds before primary closure. Wounds sustained in contaminated environments with unknown debris require thorough assessment and cleansing followed by daily reassessments to monitor for the development of infection. The use of topical antiseptics to cleanse the periwound tissue may be warranted. Patients involved in athletic, recreational, and work activities on dirt, sand, clay, or artificial playing surfaces can present with large quantities of small debris in the wound bed. Clinicians must select an appropriate technique to remove the debris while minimizing further damage to the wound bed. Wounds with clinical features of infection and adverse reactions may require more frequent cleansing because of the production of heavy exudate and the need for additional dressing changes. The production of heavy exudate can increase the risk of maceration and cause dressing saturation and leakage. Daily cleansing may be indicated to allow for clear visual inspection and assessment of the wound bed to monitor the effectiveness of topical or oral antimicrobial interventions and the progression of the infection or adverse reaction.

Clinicians should consider the frequency of cleansing in the management plan. The frequency is often debated and is based on patient, wound, and clinician needs and management plan goals. After the initial cleansing, it may not be necessary to cleanse the wound at every dressing change. Additional cleansing may be required to inspect or rehydrate the wound bed, minimize trauma to the wound bed and periwound tissue during dressing changes, promote patient comfort, and monitor infection and adverse reactions. Clinicians should not attempt to remove exudate from the wound bed through repeated cleansing in the absence of clinical features of adverse reactions or dressing integrity and barrier issues. Removing wound exudate from a clean, healthy wound may be detrimental and delay healing because exudate contains essential nutrients and growth factors.[5,14] The fluidity of the exudate allows the wound to remain moist and the nutrients and growth factors to travel to the needed areas where cells can begin the tissue repair process.[14] Healing is facilitated when there is minimal disruption to the wound bed; therefore, cleansing should only be performed when necessary.

Several clinician factors are important in selecting cleansing techniques and solutions. The skills required to perform cleansing techniques are obtained through professional training, and clinicians should become proficient with the techniques before use in the management plan. Clinicians must also possess knowledge of the anatomy of tissue; the wound healing process; and technique and solution purposes, benefits, and risks. In some settings, clinicians may need approval from institutions and organizations before using syringes, needle hubs, and plastic cannulas for irrigation. Understanding the indications and contraindications of cleansing techniques and solutions is critical to lessen the risk of adverse reactions and achieve healing outcomes.

CLEANSING TECHNIQUES

There are a variety of wound cleansing techniques that clinicians can consider for the management of acute skin trauma. The commonly used techniques among acute wounds include irrigation, showering, scrubbing and swabbing, and hydrotherapy. Cleansing is performed after the assessment of the patient and the evaluation of patient, wound, frequency, and clinician factors to combine the appropriate technique with an appropriate solution. Standard precautions and organizational policies should guide cleansing interventions, cleaning and disinfection of supplies and equipment, disposal of medical waste, and handling contaminated laundry. See Chapter 2 for further discussion on infection control and procedures. The clean technique is used for wound cleansing interventions. After a clean treatment area is prepared, the clinician should gather the appropriate supplies and equipment (Table 3-1) based on the selected technique and solution and then properly place the patient in a comfortable position. Clinicians must educate the patient on the cleansing intervention and solution to promote understanding of the goals and rationale to promote adherence to the management plan.

Irrigation

Irrigation is the process of delivering a steady flow of solution across the wound surface to remove excess secretions and loose debris and decrease bacterial contamination of the wound.[10,15] Irrigation is considered one of the most effective cleansing methods, and many have accepted wound irrigation as the standard of care.[16] This cleansing method supports wound healing while removing debris with minimal trauma to the wound bed. Clinicians must deliver the appropriate solution to the wound bed at an appropriate pressure.

Table 3-1. Supplies and Equipment for Cleansing Interventions

- Clean, boxed examination gloves
- Clean personal protective equipment
- Clean towels or linens
- Biohazard container
- Cleaning solutions and disinfectants
- Normal saline
- Potable tap water
- Topical antiseptics
- 35-mL syringe
- 18- to 20-gauge needle hub or plastic cannula
- Clean basins and cups
- Surgical sponge
- Surgical scrub brush
- Nonwoven sterile gauze

Indications

Irrigation is indicated for superficial- to full-thickness abrasions, avulsions, blisters, incisions, lacerations, and punctures. This technique is appropriate for the initial cleansing and additional cleansing when necessary.

Contraindications

Irrigation should not be performed on wounds that are actively bleeding or with wounds that expose tendons, nerves, muscles, blood vessels, or bone. If the depth or borders of a wound cannot be determined because of the development of a **tunnel**, clinicians must exercise caution with irrigation pressures to avoid forcing microorganisms or debris further into the wound or other body spaces.[15] Gentle irrigation with puncture wounds is also necessary to avoid pushing contaminants further into the cavity.

Procedures

Irrigation between the pressure range of 4 and 15 pounds per square inch (psi; 27.58-103.4 kPa) is recommended for acute skin trauma.[2,10,12,17-20] Higher pressures may cause damage to healthy granulation tissue, and lower pressures, less than 4 psi (27.58 kPa), may serve to moisten the wound bed but are unable to remove debris. A 35-mL syringe with an 18- to 20-gauge needle hub or plastic cannula (Figure 3-1) will deliver a solution to the wound bed in the pressure range of 7 to 11 psi (48.26-75.84 kPa).[2,10,11] Detailed instructions for irrigation are provided in Table 3-2. A concern with irrigation is the potential for splash back and transmitting infectious agents to patients, personnel, and the facility. Several techniques can reduce the risk of contamination, infection, and transmission of microorganisms. When using the clean technique with noninfected wounds, 2 methods lessen splash back during irrigation. After filling the syringe, place the syringe into position over the wound bed. Cup the nonsyringe hand and place just above the wound (Figure 3-5). As the syringe is depressed, adjust the cupped hand to block the solution splash back. Syringe splash guards can

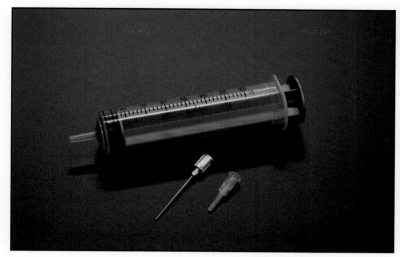

Figure 3-1. A 35-mL syringe and 19-gauge needle hub and plastic cannula.

also be purchased and used. Do not touch the wound bed with the cupped hand or splash guard. Clinicians can also use a clean, paper or plastic cup to lessen splash back. Cut a hole in the bottom of the cup with clean scissors and then fill the syringe and insert the needle hub or cannula and distal syringe through the hole in the cup. Hold the cup with the nonsyringe hand and perform irrigation (Figure 3-6). Do not allow the cup to touch the wound bed.

Showering

Showering is the use of a standard home or locker-room shower head to deliver potable tap water to the wound bed. The tap water should be from a properly treated supply and delivered through functional plumbing.

Indications

Showering can be used for superficial- to full-thickness abrasions, avulsions, blisters, lacerations, punctures, and traumatic and postoperative incisions. The technique is effective for cleansing larger, traumatic wounds.

Contraindications

Some consider wound cleansing with showering challenging because the showerhead pressure is difficult to control, and obtaining the optimal pressure in the recommended range of 4 to 15 psi (27.58-103.42 kPa) is questionable. The appropriate water temperature is also necessary to maintain an optimal healing environment.

Procedures

Turn on the shower and run the showerhead to achieve a tap water temperature between 98.6°F and 107.6°F (37°C and 42°C). The patient rinses the wound bed with tap water until all visible debris and nonviable tissue are removed. After showering, the body is dried with clean towels and the periwound tissue with sterile gauze.

Table 3-2. Wound Irrigation on a Wound Model

- Fill a clean basin with normal saline or potable tap water at a temperature between 98.6°F and 107.6°F (37°C and 42°C).
- Using a 35-mL syringe with an 18- to 20-gauge needle hub or plastic cannula, fill the syringe with normal saline or potable tap water (Figure 3-2).

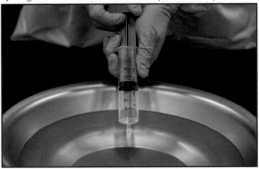

Figure 3-2

- Position the needle hub or plastic cannula tip 4 to 6 inches from the wound bed (Figure 3-3).

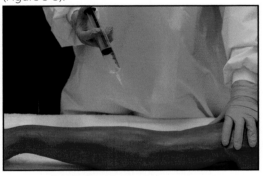

Figure 3-3

- Depress the syringe plunger with one hand and slowly sweep across the wound bed (Figure 3-4). Focus the irrigation stream over visible debris and nonviable tissue to loosen the waste. Minimize splash back with a cupped hand or cup.

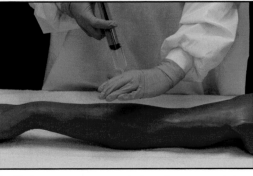

Figure 3-4

- Refill the syringe as needed and continue irrigation until all visible debris and nonviable tissue is removed.
- After irrigation, pat the periwound tissue dry with sterile gauze.

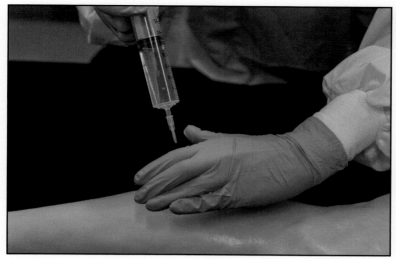

Figure 3-5. A cupped hand to block splash back from irrigation.

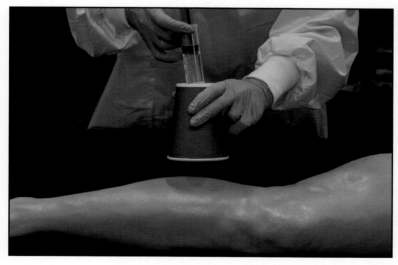

Figure 3-6. A cup to block splash back from irrigation.

Scrubbing and Swabbing

Scrubbing and swabbing is the application of a mechanical force across the wound bed with a surgical sponge; surgical scrub brush; or nonwoven, sterile gauze. This technique has been shown to remove bacteria from the wound bed, although it has not demonstrated a decrease in the incidence of infection.[2]

Indications

Scrubbing and swabbing can be used with superficial- to partial-thickness abrasions, avulsions, blisters, incisions, and lacerations contaminated with excessive debris. Clinicians may consider the technique if irrigation fails to remove debris from the wound bed. Clinicians must evaluate the benefit of removing debris with a mechanical force with the risk of damaging tissue. The scrubbing and swabbing technique is appropriate for cleansing the periwound tissue. The foam, brush, or sterile gauze should not contact the wound bed to lessen the risk of contamination.

Figure 3-7. Scrubbing with sterile gauze on a wound model.

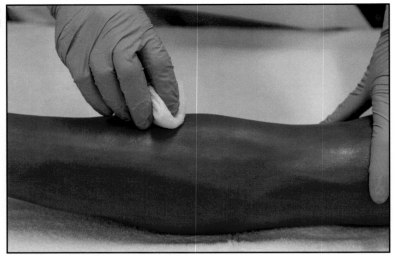

Contraindications

The scrubbing and swabbing technique is not recommended for cleansing acute skin trauma. Although the technique has demonstrated efficacy in lowering bacterial counts, scrubbing and swabbing redistributes bacteria over the wound, disrupting healing[5]; damages granulation tissue from the mechanical force; and produces an inflammatory response from shedding of gauze fibers. Scrubbing and swabbing should not be used if the wound is actively bleeding.

Procedures

Premoisten the sponge, brush, or sterile gauze with normal saline or potable tap water. The clinician often starts in the center of the wound bed, scrubbing or swabbing toward the perimeter of the wound bed in a circular pattern until the border is reached (Figure 3-7).[21] Clinicians should not bring the foam, brush, or gauze back to the center of the wound from the perimeter because this could increase the risk of contamination. The clinician should apply minimal mechanical pressure to the wound bed during the technique to lower the risk of damage to the tissues. The technique is completed with the removal of the visible debris from the wound bed. For the periwound tissue, premoisten the sponge, brush, or sterile gauze with normal saline, potable tap water, or topical antiseptic. The clinician remains outside the wound perimeter and scrubs or swabs the periwound tissue. Clinicians should avoid foam, brush, or gauze contact with the wound bed.

Hydrotherapy

Whirlpool baths are a common method of hydrotherapy, and although considered a cleansing technique, whirlpool baths are more frequently used for the debridement of chronic wounds.[22,23] Whirlpool baths remove gross contaminants and debris and hydrate the wound bed through immersion in potable tap water. Another form of hydrotherapy sometimes used in athletic training facilities is soaking the wound in a plastic basin or tub of potable tap water.

Indications

Hydrotherapy can be used on superficial- to full-thickness wounds with eschar, heavy contamination of debris, and loosely adherent necrotic tissue. Hydrotherapy may also be used with other cleansing techniques, such as irrigation, to remove debris from the wound bed.

Contraindications

Hydrotherapy used as the sole cleansing technique for acute skin trauma is not recommended.[2] Although hydrotherapy effectively removes wound contaminants and debris in the inflammatory phase of healing,[2] clinicians must consider the adverse effects of the technique. When an agitator or turbine is used, it is difficult to control the pressure of the tap water delivered to the wound bed. Higher pressures generated can damage developing granulation tissue, hinder migrating epidermal cells and neutrophils, and cause maceration of the wound bed and periwound tissue.[10,24,25] The use of an agitator is not recommended when new granulating and epithelializing tissue is present.[10,24-26] Soaking in a basin or tub disrupts the moisture balance of the wound bed and is not considered an appropriate cleansing technique for acute skin trauma.[10] Hydrotherapy has been associated with wound infection; this is more commonly seen in the hospital environment.[24] Based on the increased risk of infection, topical antiseptic solutions are often added to tap water during treatment. The clinician must consider the benefits of using antiseptic solutions to control bacteria and lessen the risk of infection while potentially impeding tissue healing because of the cytotoxic effects of the solutions. Clinicians must also strictly follow infection control policies and procedures for cleaning and disinfecting whirlpool tubs and plastic basins or tubs after each patient to lessen the risk of cross-contamination.[25]

Procedures

The body part and wound are submerged in a whirlpool tub filled with potable tap water between 92.0°F and 96.0°F (33.3°C and 35.5°C) for 10 to 20 minutes.[24] The water temperature and immersion time for soaking in a basin or tub vary among clinicians. After hydrotherapy, the body part is dried with clean towels and the periwound tissue with sterile gauze. Irrigation can be performed if additional cleansing is necessary.

CLEANSING SOLUTIONS

In addition to selecting the most appropriate technique, selecting an appropriate nontoxic solution to remove debris and create the optimal healing environment is essential. Selecting a wound cleansing solution is as critical as the chosen technique. Several solutions are available for cleansing acute skin trauma. The optimal cleansing solution should be nontoxic to human tissue, remain effective in the presence of organic material, reduce the number of microorganisms, not cause a sensitivity reaction, be widely available, and be cost-effective.[27] The solution should be effective against the bacterial flora in the wound yet not inhibit or damage the cells involved in the healing process.[28] Common cleansing solutions for acute wounds include normal saline, potable tap water, and topical antiseptics. Clinicians must consider patient, wound, and clinician factors in the selection of an appropriate solution and technique. Clinicians should carefully evaluate the potential harms and benefits of the available solutions and techniques in the management plan to achieve healing outcomes.

Figure 3-8. A normal saline solution bottle.

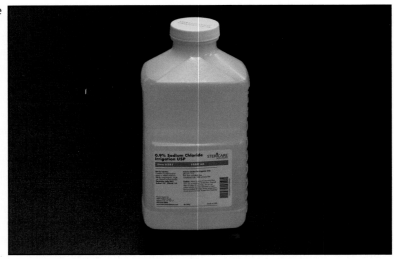

Figure 3-9. Normal saline solution ampoules.

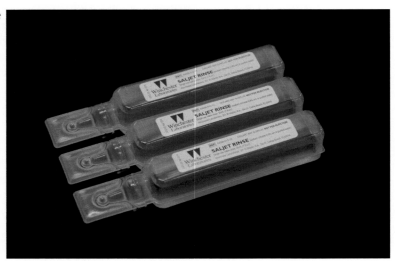

Normal Saline and Potable Tap Water

Normal saline and potable tap water are the preferred cleansing solutions for acute skin trauma. These solutions are most effective when combined with irrigation for cleansing the wound bed. Normal saline is an isotonic solution and does not draw from or add fluid to the wound bed. Normal saline may also be more effective in maintaining the moisture balance in the wound bed. Normal saline is available in various containers and is commonly purchased in bottles (Figure 3-8) and ampoules (Figure 3-9). Potable tap water from a properly treated supply and plumbing system is considered a safe alternative for cleansing acute skin trauma. Some suggest that potable water from the tap should run for a couple of minutes to clear standing water and rid the supply of any impurities. A referral is warranted in wounds with exposed bone, tendon, muscle, nerve, or blood vessels, and advanced cleansing with normal saline is usually performed.[13]

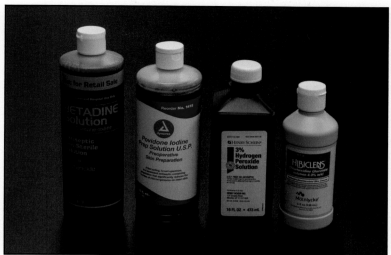

Figure 3-10. Topical antiseptics.

Topical Antiseptics

Topical antiseptics are antimicrobial agents used to eradicate or decrease the number of microorganisms in the wound bed or periwound tissue.[20,29,30] The commonly used topical antiseptics for cleansing acute skin trauma include povidone-iodine, hydrogen peroxide, and chlorhexidine gluconate (Figure 3-10). Antiseptics have been used for cleansing acute wounds to prevent and manage infection for many years. However, the use of antiseptics has generated much controversy based on their cytotoxicity to tissues. Antiseptic solutions have cytotoxic effects on fibroblasts, keratinocytes, and other vital wound healing components.[31,32] These solutions cause delayed wound healing and reduced wound strength. As a result of these concerns, some clinicians may opt to dilute the antiseptic to reduce the high cytotoxicity.[28] Although diluted solutions may not be as toxic as the undiluted forms, determining a safe level of diluted concentration that is effective against bacteria and not harmful to tissue is challenging. Topical antiseptics can safely be used to cleanse the periwound tissue in diluted and undiluted forms. Clinicians should avoid direct contact of the antiseptic with the wound bed when healthy, granulating tissue is present. Clinicians must weigh the benefits of using antiseptic solutions against the resultant damage and trauma to the wound bed.[28] Topical antiseptics for infection prophylaxis should be considered for wounds with developing clinical features of infection, debris or nonviable tissue contamination of unknown origins, and delayed reporting and assessment.[29] Clinicians should use caution in the routine use of topical antiseptics in uncomplicated acute skin trauma and base selection and use on the purposes and goals of the management plan.

CLEANSING SOLUTION TEMPERATURE

Clinicians should also consider the temperature of the solution delivered to the wound bed with the cleansing intervention. Most recommend a solution temperature between 98.6°F and 107.6°F (37°C and 42°C).[8,9,33,34] Optimal cellular activity is achieved when the temperature of the wound bed remains at 98.6°F (37°C). Lower temperatures result in less oxygen and fewer leukocytes, fibroblasts, and macrophages in the wound bed, delaying the healing process.[29,33] A reduction in the temperature of the wound bed can also result during patient reassessments with frequent cleansing and dressing changes. Unnecessary exposure to cooler temperatures caused by cold cleansing solutions and frequent dressing changes will alter the wound bed temperature and interfere with **mitotic activity**. After a cold solution is applied, it can take up to 40 minutes for the wound to return to the optimal temperature for healing.[33] Clinicians should ensure that cleansing of the wound bed is warranted, and an appropriate temperature of the solution is maintained to lessen the risk of adverse outcomes.[29]

SUMMARY OF EVIDENCE

Limited evidence-based medicine reviews and clinical investigations have examined the effectiveness of cleansing techniques and solutions on the rates of infection and healing in the management of acute skin trauma. Irrigation is considered the preferred method of wound cleansing. An evidence-based medicine review reported reduced rates of infection and inflammation among acute and chronic wounds irrigated with a pressure of 13 psi (89.63 kPa).[11] However, an agreement on the optimal pressure for irrigation to create an environment conducive for healing is needed. The authors of a separate review examined the efficacy of irrigation and swabbing with normal saline among acute and chronic wounds healing by secondary intention.[16] Only one trial met the inclusion criteria and demonstrated irrigation with pressures from 4 to 13 psi (27.58-89.63 kPa), reduced rates of infection and patient pain, and increased rates of healing and was cost-effective compared to scrubbing.

The effects of showering on the rates of infection and healing and the timing of the intervention have been examined in several evidence-based reviews. A 2012 Cochrane review examining showering vs no showering among patients with postoperative lacerations and incisions revealed no differences in the rates of infection and healing.[12] This 2012 review[12] was updated,[35] and the quasi-randomized trials investigating the effects of showering were excluded based on updates to the review methodology. Debate exists over the timing of when showering can be used for incisions, and it is a common question among postoperative patients. Many patients are instructed to keep the incision dry for 48 hours when skin re-epithelialization has occurred.[36,37] The authors of an evidence-based review reported no increase in the rates of infection and complications among postoperative incisions between showering within 48 hours and beyond 3 days.[37] A separate evidence-based review included one trial and examined the effects of showering within 12 hours and after 48 hours among postoperative sutured excisional wounds.[38] The findings demonstrated no conclusive evidence for differences in the rates of infection between early and delayed postoperative showering. It is important to recognize that early showering has not been associated with an increase in the rate of infection or delayed healing. Clinicians should consider the psychological benefit of early showering because overall patient satisfaction and well-being are often improved.[12]

Multiple evidence-based medicine reviews have examined the efficacy of normal saline and potable tap water on the rates of infection and healing among various acute and chronic wounds.[35,39,40] A 2009 review found tap water produced lower rates of infection compared with normal saline.[40] In a 2014 review, the authors reported no differences in the rates of infection and healing between normal saline and potable tap water.[39] The authors concluded that normal saline or potable tap water can be safely used as solutions to cleanse acute wounds.[39,40] A 2022 Cochrane review reported no clear evidence to determine the effects of normal saline and potable tap water on the rates of infection and healing.[35] Individual trials included in the review comparing normal saline and potable tap water demonstrated no differences in the rates of infection and healing.[35] Two trials in the review revealed tap water was cost-effective as a cleansing solution compared with normal saline.[35] There are frequently cited findings from a clinical investigation that favor potable tap water over normal saline for cleansing of traumatic lacerations.[41] In this investigation, the authors reported lower rates of infection in wounds cleansed with potable tap water.[41] However, there was a difference in the temperature of the solutions; the potable tap water was at 98.6°F (37°C), and the normal saline was at room temperature. This temperature difference may have contributed to the efficacy of potable tap water among the traumatic lacerations. Despite the evidence that supports both normal saline and potable tap water as effective cleansing solutions, potable tap water is still not used universally in clinical practice.[29]

There continues to be disagreement in the literature surrounding the use of topical antiseptics in the management of acute skin trauma. Numerous studies have reported conflicting results on the bactericidal effects and cytotoxicity of topical antiseptics, including povidone-iodine, hydrogen peroxide, and chlorhexidine. Some findings demonstrate the impairment of wound healing and minimal effects against bacteria, whereas others show improved wound healing and bactericidal effectiveness.[11,28,30,32,42] Most agree that topical antiseptics can be safely used to disinfect the periwound tissue. Investigations examining the effects of topical antiseptics on the wound bed are inconclusive. After adequate cleansing and in the later stages of wound healing, topical antiseptics such as povidone-iodine may have some benefit on heavily colonized or infected wounds.[8] There is moderate evidence to suggest that irrigating contaminated wounds with 1% povidone-iodine reduces infection rates, whereas soaking with 1% povidone-iodine did not reduce bacterial counts.[11]

SUMMARY

Cleansing acute skin trauma is essential to promote healing and reduce the risk of infection and adverse reactions. Appropriate techniques and solutions remove debris, exudate, microorganisms, and nonviable waste from the wound bed and periwound tissue. Cleansing interventions create a clean, moist, and warm wound environment; allow visual assessment of the wound bed; return moisture to the wound bed; and provide patients with a sense of well-being. Patient health status and preferences, wound characteristics, infection and adverse reactions, cleansing frequency, and clinician knowledge and experience will guide the selection of an appropriate technique and solution. Clinicians can consider irrigation, showering, scrubbing and swabbing, and hydrotherapy as cleansing techniques. Solutions available to clinicians include normal saline, potable tap water, and topical antiseptics. The temperature of the solution is critical to avoid disrupting the healing process. Clinicians should carefully consider the risks and benefits of the cleansing techniques and solutions and the frequency of cleansing to support the goals of the management plan.

REFERENCES

1. Luedtke-Hoffmann KA, Schafer DS. Pulsed lavage in wound cleansing. *Phys Ther.* 2000;80(3):292-300.

2. Barr JE. Principles of wound cleansing. *Ostomy Wound Manage.* 1995;41(7A suppl):15S-21S.

3. Rodeheaver GT. Pressure ulcer debridement and cleansing: A review of current literature. *Ostomy Wound Manage.* 1999;45:80S-85S.

4. Carr M. Wound cleansing: Sorely neglected? *Prim Intention.* 2006;14(4):150-161.

5. Towler J. Cleansing traumatic wounds with swabs, water or saline. *J Wound Care.* 2001;10(6):231-234.

6. Wynn M. The benefits and harms of cleansing for acute traumatic wounds: A narrative review. *Adv Skin Wound Care.* 2021;34(9):488-492.

7. Blunt J. Wound cleansing: Ritualistic or research-based practice? *Nurs Stand.* 2001;16(1):33-36.

8. Fletcher J. Wound cleansing. *Prof Nurse.* 1997;12(11):793-796.

9. Davies C. Wound care. Cleansing rites and wrongs. *Nurs Times.* 1999;95(43):71-72, 75.

10. Nicks BA, Ayello EA, Woo K, Nitzki-George D, Sibbald RG. Acute wound management: Revisiting the approach to assessment, irrigation, and closure considerations. *Int J Emerg Med.* 2010;3(4):399-407.

11. Fernandez R, Griffiths R, Ussia C. Effectiveness of solutions, techniques and pressure in wound cleansing. *JBI Reports.* 2004;2(7):231-270.

12. Fernandez R, Griffiths R. Water for wound cleansing. *Cochrane Database Syst Rev.* 2012;2:CD003861.

13. Lindholm C, Bergsten A, Berglund E. Chronic wounds and nursing care. *J Wound Care.* 1999;8(1):5-10.

14. Adderley UJ. Managing wound exudate and promoting healing. *Br J Community Nurs.* 2010;15:S15-S20.

15. Lewis K, Pay JL. *Wound Irrigation.* StatPearls Publishing; 2023.

16. Rajhathy E, Vander Meer J, Valenzano T, et al. Wound irrigation versus swabbing technique for cleansing non-infected chronic wounds: A systematic review of differences in bleeding, pain, infection, exudate and necrotic tissue. *J Tissue Viability.* 2023;32(1):136-143. doi: 10.1016/j.jtv.2022.11.002.

17. Pressure ulcer treatment. Agency for Health Care Policy and Research. *Clin Pract Guidel Quick Ref Guide Clin.* 1994;15:1-25.

18. Rodeheaver GT, Pettry D, Thacker JG, Edgerton MT, Edlich RF. Wound cleansing by high pressure irrigation. *Surg Gynecol Obstet.* 1975;141(3):357-362.

19. Cunliffe PJ, Fawcett TN. Wound cleansing: The evidence for the techniques and solutions used. *Prof Nurse.* 2002;18(2):95-99.

20. Atiyeh BS, Dibo SA, Hayek SN. Wound cleansing, topical antiseptics and wound healing. *Int Wound J.* 2009;6(6):420-430.

21. Myers BA. *Wound Management: Principles and Practice.* 2nd ed. Pearson Prentice Hall; 2008:70-93.

22. Albaugh K, Loehne H. Wound bed preparation/débridement. In: McCulloch JM, Kloth LC, eds. *Wound Healing: Evidence-Based Management.* 4th ed. F.A. Davis; 2010:155-179.

23. Myers BA. *Wound Management: Principles and Practice.* 2nd ed. Pearson Prentice Hall; 2008:160-195.

24. Tao H, Butler JP, Luttrell T. The role of whirlpool in wound care. *J Am Coll Clin Wound Spec.* 2013;4(1):7-12.

25. Hess CL, Howard MA, Attinger CE. A review of mechanical adjuncts in wound healing: Hydrotherapy, ultrasound, negative pressure therapy, hyperbaric oxygen, and electrostimulation. *Ann Plast Surg.* 2003;51(2):210-218.

26. Trevelyan J. Wound cleansing: Principles and practice. *Nurs Times.* 1996;92(16):46-48.

27. Flanagan M. Wound cleansing. In: Morrison M, Moffatt C, Bridel-Nixon J, Bale S, eds. *Nursing Management of Chronic Wounds.* C.V. Mosby Co; 1997:87-102.

28. Rabenberg VS, Ingersoll CD, Sandrey MA, Johnson MT. The bactericidal and cytotoxic effects of antimicrobial wound cleansers. *J Athl Train.* 2002;37(1):51-54.

29. Brown A. When is wound cleansing necessary and what solution should be used? *Nurs Times.* 2018;114(9):40.

30. Kramer SA. Effect of povidone-iodine on wound healing: A review. *J Vasc Nurs.* 1999;17(1):17-23.

31. Lineaweaver W, Howard R, Soucy D, et al. Topical antimicrobial toxicity. *Arch Surg.* 1985;120(3):267-270.

32. Drosou A, Falabella A, Kirsner RS. Antiseptics on wounds: An area of controversy. *Wounds.* 2003;15(5):149-166.

33. Lock PM. The effects of temperature on mitotic activity at the edge of experimental wounds. In: Lundgren A, Soner AB, eds. *Symposia on Wound Healing: Plastic Surgical and Dermatological Aspects.* 1980.

34. Watret L, Armitage M. Making sense of wound cleansing. *J Community Nurs.* 2002;16(4):27-34.

35. Fernandez R, Green HL, Griffiths R, Atkinson RA, Ellwood LJ. Water for wound cleansing. *Cochrane Database Syst Rev.* 2022;9:CD003861.

36. Yu AL, Alfieri DC, Bartucci KN, Holzmeister AM, Rees HW. Wound hygiene practices after total knee arthroplasty: Does it matter? *J Arthroplasty.* 2016;31(10):2256-2259.

37. Copeland-Halperin L, Reategui Via y Rada, Maria L, et al. Does the timing of postoperative showering impact infection rates? A systematic review and meta-analysis. *J Plast Reconstr Aesthet Surg.* 2020;73(7):1306-1311.

38. Toon CD, Sinha S, Davidson BR, Gurusamy KS. Early versus delayed post-operative bathing or showering to prevent wound complications. *Cochrane Database Syst Rev.* 2015;7:CD010075.

39. Queirós P, Santos E, Apóstolo J, Cardoso D, Cunha M, Rodrigues M. The effectiveness of cleansing solutions for wound treatment: A systematic review. *JBI Database Syst Rev Implement Rep.* 2014;12(10):121-151.

40. Bee TS, Maniya S, Fang ZR, et al. Wound bed preparation—Cleansing techniques and solutions: A systematic review. *Singapore Nurs J.* 2009;36(1):16-22.

41. Angerås MH, Brandberg A, Falk A, Seeman T. Comparison between sterile saline and tap water for the cleaning of acute traumatic soft tissue wounds. *Eur J Surg.* 1992;158(6-7):347-350.

42. Vermeulen H, Westerbos SJ, Ubbink DT. Benefit and harm of iodine in wound care: A systematic review. *J Hosp Infect.* 2010;76(3):191-199.

4

DEBRIDEMENT

The overall goal in the management of acute skin trauma is to create a moist, clean, and warm environment to promote healing. Debridement of the wound bed is considered a standard clinical practice to achieve healing outcomes. After cleansing, some acute wounds may require debridement to create an optimal healing environment and prepare the wound for the application of a dressing. Debridement is the removal of traumatized, necrotic tissue, foreign debris (eg, sand, grass, and/or dirt), and microorganisms from the wound bed that can impede normal healing. This chapter provides an overview of the debridement techniques used to manage acute skin trauma. The chapter begins with a discussion on the goal and purposes of debridement. Next, patient, wound, and clinician factors for technique selection are presented. The chapter concludes with individual debridement techniques, including indications, contraindications, and procedures, for acute wounds.

DEBRIDEMENT GOAL AND PURPOSES

After a thorough cleansing, debridement is used to create an environment conducive for healing. The goal is to debride the wound bed until only normal vascularized tissue remains, creating a viable wound bed for the progression of normal healing.[1] A viable wound is represented with red

DOI: 10.1201/9781003523055-4

granulation tissue covering the wound bed. The purposes of debridement are to remove necrotic tissue and foreign material from the wound bed. Necrotic tissue left on the wound bed can delay healing and serve as a medium for the growth of microorganisms.[2] Debridement of traumatized tissue decreases the bacterial bioburden and allows the body's endogenous enzymes to digest the remaining necrotic tissue, lessening the risk of infection.[2,3] The body's defense mechanism and natural debridement slow with the presence of necrotic tissue in the wound. Debridement improves the function of leukocytes, supporting the body's defense and reducing the risk of infection.[4,5] Necrotic tissue and foreign material can delay healing by prolonging the inflammatory phase and creating a barrier to the growth of new tissue. The inflammatory phase and removal of cellular debris and microorganisms are shortened with debridement, decreasing the energy required for the progression of normal healing.[5,6] A viable, vascularized wound bed produced by debridement allows an unobstructed environment for epithelial cells to migrate across the wound surface and achieve wound contraction.[4]

FACTORS TO CONSIDER FOR DEBRIDEMENT

Clinical decisions regarding the debridement of acute skin trauma are based on several factors. The clinician must consider the health status of the patient, characteristics of the wound, their level of knowledge and experience with debridement techniques, and applicable state practice acts to determine whether debridement is necessary and which technique to use.[4] The patient's medical history and status are factors to consider before debridement. For example, autolytic debridement should not be considered if the patient is allergic to materials used in occlusive dressings. Comorbidities that contribute to a delay in healing and the development of infection can influence technique selection. Mechanical debridement techniques (eg, wet to dry, scrubbing, and hydrotherapy) can produce pain and are inappropriate for patients with a low threshold. The clinician should fully explain the debridement technique and goals to develop patient adherence to the management plan.

Several wound factors are critical in selecting an appropriate debridement technique. Clinicians must consider wound etiology, type and color of the tissue, presence of foreign debris, and clinical features of infection or adverse reactions. The mechanism, time, and location of injury can predict the amount of tissue damage, contamination, and condition of the wound bed.[7] Wounds caused by shear force, such as abrasions and blisters, may contain denuded or necrotic tissue within the wound bed or attached to the wound border. A patient who delays reporting a wound may present with black, hard eschar adhered to the wound bed or perimeter. Wounds sustained on athletic playing surfaces can contain foreign debris (eg, dirt, sand, grass, and/or crumb rubber pellets) in varying amounts. These wounds may require debridement after cleansing to remove necrotic tissue, foreign debris, and microorganisms. Clinicians should exercise caution in the debridement of wounds that demonstrate viable, red granulation tissue after cleansing. Debridement of the granular surface can cause further damage and delay healing. Debridement of wounds with clinical features of infection and adverse reactions can be performed and warrant referral for further evaluation. See the individual debridement techniques in the following section for indications and contraindications.

Clinicians should also consider their knowledge and skill level in determining debridement methods. Competence with all aspects of the management plan, including debridement, is required to promote healing and lessen adverse outcomes. Knowledge of the anatomy of tissue and the ability to differentiate between viable and nonviable tissue are necessary to prevent further damage to the wound.[2] The clinician should use only those debridement techniques in which they have received professional training, are comfortable performing, and have access to adequate supplies and equipment. Some methods of debridement may be restricted to specific health care professions. Clinicians should review applicable state practice acts to verify.[8]

Table 4-1. Supplies and Equipment for Debridement Interventions

- Sterile instruments (eg, scissors, forceps, and tweezers)
- Clean scissors
- Clean, boxed examination gloves
- Clean personal protective equipment
- Clean towels or linens
- Biohazard container
- Cleaning solutions and disinfectants
- Normal saline
- Potable tap water
- Topical antiseptics
- 35-mL syringe
- 18- to 20-gauge needle hub or plastic cannula
- Clean basins and cups
- Surgical scrub brush
- High-porosity sponge
- Occlusive dressings (eg, alginates, films, foams, hydrogels, and hydrocolloids)
- Woven and nonwoven sterile gauze
- Woven sterile gauze with large pores

DEBRIDEMENT TECHNIQUES

There are many debridement methods available to the clinician in the management of acute skin trauma. The techniques that clinicians can consider are autolytic, conservative sharp, irrigation, scrubbing, wet-to-dry, wet-to-moist, hydrotherapy, and chemical debridement. Debridement is performed after the cleansing of the wound bed and assessment of the patient, wound, and clinician factors. Clinicians should follow standard precautions and organizational policies during debridement interventions, cleaning and disinfection, disposal of medical waste, and handling contaminated laundry. See Chapter 2 for further discussion of infection control procedures. The clean technique is appropriate for the debridement of acute skin trauma. The clinician should prepare a clean treatment area, gather the necessary equipment and supplies (Table 4-1), and comfortably position the patient for the debridement intervention. Patient education on the debridement intervention can promote understanding and adherence to the overall management plan.

Autolytic Debridement

Autolytic debridement is the use of the body's mechanisms to soften, liquefy, and digest necrotic or devitalized tissue and waste. In a warm, moist wound environment, neutrophils, macrophages, and phagocytic cells digest tissue and waste through the release of endogenous proteolytic and collagenolytic enzymes.[2,3] The moist environment is created by the application of semipermeable or impermeable occlusive dressings such as alginates, films, foams, hydrogels, and hydrocolloids.[2-4,6] Autolytic debridement is the most conservative and time-consuming debridement technique, occurring over several days.[2-4,6] The technique results in minimal pain, requires knowledge of occlusive dressing indications and contraindications, and is consistent with moist wound healing.[4,6]

Figure 4-1. Autolytic debridement with a hydrocolloid dressing.

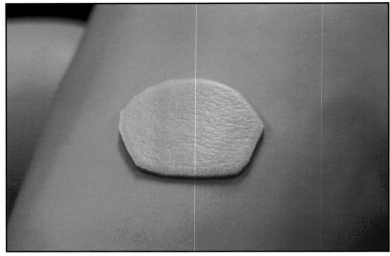

Indications

Autolytic debridement is indicated for superficial- to full-thickness abrasions, avulsions, incisions, and lacerations; superficial- to full-thickness blisters after the removal of the devitalized roof with conservative sharp debridement[9]; and superficial- to partial-thickness punctures.[5] Autolytic debridement is commonly used with irrigation, wet-to-moist, or conservative sharp debridement methods for selective removal of the remaining necrotic tissue. Autolytic debridement is also useful for patients who cannot tolerate other forms of debridement or when monitoring and reassessments are infrequent, with patient education provided.[2]

Contraindications

Autolytic debridement should not be used with clinically infected wounds.[3,6] The technique should be discontinued immediately if signs and symptoms of infection are suspected.[6] Desiccated wounds do not support autolytic debridement until moisture is trapped and managed over the wound bed under an occlusive dressing.[3]

Procedures

The semipermeable or impermeable dressing is applied over the wound bed and adhered to the periwound tissue (Figure 4-1). The dressing remains over the wound bed for consecutive days based on the dressing selected. Clinicians should monitor and reassess the patient, wound, periwound tissue, and dressing daily for adverse reactions. Reassessment of the wound bed is influenced by the dressing applied because some dressings do not allow for visual inspection while over the wound. Clinicians should avoid unnecessary dressing changes for wound bed inspection in an asymptomatic patient. Autolytic debridement will result in the normal production of fluid or gel over the wound bed. The fluid is brownish, can have a foul odor, and should not be mistaken for infection.[10-12] Irrigation can be used to remove the fluid and liquefied waste with dressing changes to assess the wound bed. Autolytic debridement is slow and may require multiple dressings to remove the tissue and waste.[6] When the wound is free of necrotic tissue and waste through autolytic debridement, occlusive dressings can maintain a moist wound environment until complete healing.[4]

Conservative Sharp Debridement

Conservative sharp debridement is the removal of loosely adherent devitalized tissue that lies superficial to viable tissue with sterile scissors, forceps, and tweezers.[2,9] Acute skin trauma should be debrided of all necrotic or devitalized, nonbleeding tissue as soon as possible to lessen the risk of infection and to promote healing.[1] Clinicians must review state laws and practice acts to determine the use of sharp instruments and the technique.[8]

Indications

Conservative sharp debridement can be used with superficial- to full-thickness abrasions, avulsions, blisters, incisions, and lacerations with loosely adhered devitalized tissue.[6,13] Conservative sharp debridement is a selective technique removing only devitalized tissue without trauma to viable tissue. Unlike sharp techniques for chronic wounds, conservative sharp debridement of acute skin trauma is typically performed in a single visit.[13] Following the technique, autolytic debridement can be used to remove any remaining devitalized tissue and promote a moist wound environment.

Contraindications

Conservative sharp debridement requires knowledge of anatomical structures and tissue types, proficiency with sharp instruments, and approval from state practice acts before performing.[2,6,9] Conservative sharp debridement is contraindicated when the structures or tissues cannot be identified; when a border between nonviable and viable tissue cannot be visualized; when the patient is not comfortable with the technique; when the clinician is not confident in their skill and experience; or when appropriate supplies, equipment, and management setting are not accessible.[4]

Procedures

Clinicians should carefully consider the preparation and performance of conservative sharp debridement based on the use of sharp instruments.[4] The sterile scissors, forceps, and tweezers should be high quality in disposable or reusable forms. Suture removal kits are not designed to cut devitalized tissue and should not be used.[1,2] Clinicians should carefully examine the wound bed to identify the type and color of the tissue. Loosely adherent devitalized or necrotic tissue is white or tan compared to red, viable granulation tissue. The clinician should determine whether a border exists between nonviable and viable tissue.[1,14] With a clear and visible border, the nonviable tissue is gently lifted with forceps or tweezers and then cut with scissors along the border, leaving a thin margin of nonviable tissue intact (Figure 4-2). If nonviable tissue is identified and the border is unclear, begin at the center and cut concentric circles of nonviable tissue until viable tissue is approached. The scissors should remain parallel to the wound to avoid trauma to the underlying tissues.[4] The procedure should be performed in a slow, methodical fashion and stopped if bleeding occurs.[2] Clinicians should not attempt to remove small amounts of devitalized tissue along the border with viable tissue (Figure 4-3). Further cutting may extend into healthy tissue, causing trauma and bleeding. After the removal of as much devitalized tissue as possible, irrigate the wound with normal saline or potable tap water before applying the dressing.[2]

Closed blisters with an intact, nonviable roof affecting athletic, recreational, or work activities may require removal to allow the patient full movement and function.[8] This procedure may be considered a surgical technique in some states, and clinicians should review the regulations before performing. Cleanse the blister roof and periwound tissue by scrubbing with sterile gauze soaked with a topical antiseptic. Cut a small incision in the roof with a sharp, sterile instrument and allow the blister to drain. The incision is made away from viable tissue to avoid trauma. Using sterile instruments, remove the roof with the conservative sharp technique described previously. Closed blisters not affecting athletic, recreational, or work activities should be left intact and protected.

Figure 4-2. Conservative sharp debridement of an open blister.

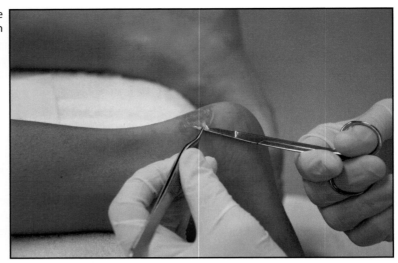

Figure 4-3. An open blister debrided with the conservative sharp technique. Devitalized tissue present on the border (white) with viable granulation tissue covering the wound bed (red).

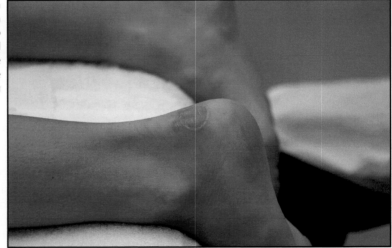

Irrigation

Irrigation is the delivery of a fluid to the wound bed to remove loosely adherent superficial debris and necrotic tissue, reduce microorganisms, and maintain a moist environment. This technique can serve as an extension of cleansing for the debridement of acute skin trauma.[5]

Indications

Irrigation is indicated for superficial- to full-thickness abrasions, avulsions, blisters, incisions, lacerations, and punctures.[3,7,15,16] This technique can be used with noninfected and infected wounds with loose debris.[2] Irrigation may be used alone or in combination with other debridement techniques to achieve a viable wound bed.

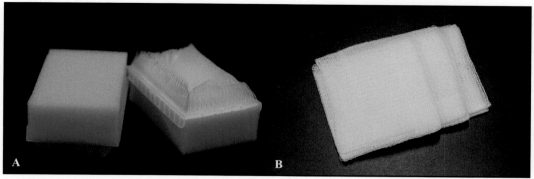

Figure 4-4. (A) Sponge/surgical scrub brush. (B) Sterile gauze.

Contraindications

Irrigation should not be used for wounds with thick, hard eschar.[2] At the recommended pressure ranges, normal saline or potable tap water is unable to penetrate and moisten the devitalized tissue to achieve debridement goals.[2] Irrigation should not be performed when profuse bleeding is present.[17]

Procedures

Irrigation for debridement purposes is identical to the irrigation procedure for cleansing discussed in Chapter 3. Normal saline or potable tap water is delivered in a constant stream to the wound bed through a 35-mL syringe with an 18- to 20-gauge needle hub or plastic cannula at pressure ranges from 4 to 15 pounds per square inch (psi; 27.58-103.4 kPa).[3,7,16,18] A lower pressure range from 2 to 4 psi (13.79-27.58 kPa) is recommended for puncture wounds to avoid driving debris, necrotic tissue, and contaminants deeper into the wound.[3,7,16,18] Tap water should not be used in wounds with exposed tendon or bone.[5] After irrigation, the periwound tissue is patted dry with sterile gauze to prepare for dressing application. Splash back is often produced during irrigation. Clinicians should use appropriate personal protective equipment and follow infection control guidelines with this technique.

Scrubbing

Scrubbing is the use of a sponge, surgical scrub brush, or sterile gauze along with a fluid to remove nonadherent necrotic tissue and debris from the wound bed (Figure 4-4).[4] A high-porosity (90 pores/square inch [14 pores/cm^2]) sponge is recommended for the technique.[4]

Indications

Scrubbing can be used with superficial- to partial-thickness abrasions, avulsions, blisters, incisions, and lacerations contaminated with large quantities of small debris (eg, sand, grass, clay, asphalt, and/or crumb rubber pellets).[4,5] Because of the heavy contamination, clinicians may select scrubbing in the immediate management of some wounds. Clinicians should carefully consider the benefits of scrubbing and mechanically removing debris from the wound bed against the potential of damage to granulation tissue.[4] Scrubbing can safely be used on the periwound tissue. Clinicians should avoid touching the wound bed with a sponge, brush, or sterile gauze to prevent possible contamination of the wound bed.

Contraindications

Scrubbing is a nonselective debridement technique and can damage or remove healthy granulation tissue. The mechanical pressure of the sponge, brush, or sterile gauze can produce pain when debriding a wound covered with granulation tissue. Aggressive pressure and friction can also cause bleeding of the wound bed.[2]

Procedures

The sponge, brush, or sterile gauze is premoistened with normal saline or potable tap water. The clinician scours the wound bed from the middle and progresses toward the wound margins in a circular pattern.[4] The clinician should apply minimal mechanical pressure to the wound during the technique to lessen the risk of trauma to tissues. Scrubbing should be terminated when the nonadherent tissue or debris is removed from the wound bed. For the periwound tissue, a sponge, brush, or sterile gauze is premoistened with normal saline, potable tap water, or topical antiseptic. The clinician scrubs the periwound tissue in a parallel pattern to the wound, avoiding contact with the wound bed.

Wet to Dry

Wet-to-dry debridement, or wet-to-dry dressing, is the application of moist sterile gauze to the wound bed. The gauze is left on the wound bed until completely dry and then quickly removed to debride necrotic tissue and foreign debris.[3] As drying occurs, the gauze adheres to the wound bed and traps necrotic tissue, exudate, and debris within the weave pattern and fibers of the gauze.[2,4] The adhered tissue and debris are removed as the gauze is lifted from the wound.[2,4]

Indications

Wet-to-dry debridement is indicated for wounds with loose, necrotic tissue that can adhere to the gauze fibers.[2] The technique can be used alone or in combination with other debridement methods. Wet-to-dry debridement can be considered when the risk of trauma to healthy, viable tissue does not exceed the benefit of mechanically removing necrotic tissue and debris from the wound bed.[2] Many suggest the use of more selective debridement techniques to lessen the risk of trauma to healthy tissues.[2,4]

Contraindications

Wet-to-dry debridement is not recommended for acute skin trauma.[5] The nonselective technique should not be used with the presence of granulation tissue in the wound bed.[2,4] Granulation tissue can adhere to and possibly grow within the gauze as the dressing and wound dehydrate.[4] Lifting the dressing from the wound bed upon drying can remove adhered granulation and necrotic tissue, causing trauma and delayed healing. Wet-to-dry debridement promotes desiccation of the wound bed, which is contradictory to the goal of a moist wound environment and promoting healing.[2,4] The technique can also increase the risk of maceration to the periwound tissue and cause pain and bleeding with dressing adherence and removal.[2]

Procedures

Woven, sterile gauze with large pores is saturated with normal saline, potable tap water, or chemicals and then squeezed until damp.[16,19] Normal saline is the preferred solution for the technique.[4,6] The gauze is placed over all surfaces of the wound bed and covered with additional dry gauze layers and a secondary dressing.[6] The gauze on the wound bed is allowed to remain in place for 8 to 24 hours until dried and adhered and then quickly lifted and removed.[4,20] If used, wet-to-dry debridement should be discontinued in a clean wound with visible, viable tissue.[16]

Wet to Moist

Wet-to-moist debridement, or wet-to-moist dressing, is the placement of moist sterile gauze over the wound bed. The gauze is left on the wound bed and removed before drying is complete.[5] Loose necrotic tissue, debris, and eschar adhere to the gauze and are removed when the dressing is lifted from the wound bed. The wet-to-moist technique is a rapid method of debridement.[5]

Indications

Wet-to-moist debridement can be used for superficial- to full-thickness abrasions, avulsions, blisters, incisions, and lacerations with loosely adherent necrotic tissue, foreign debris, and eschar.[5] The technique is often used before other debridement methods to return moisture to the wound bed, soften hard eschar, and loosen necrotic tissue and debris. Wet-to-moist dressings can be followed by irrigation, conservative sharp, or autolytic debridement to remove necrotic tissue, debris, and eschar.

Contraindications

Wet-to-moist debridement is selective in the removal of necrotic tissue and debris from the wound bed. Although the technique causes less trauma and pain with dressing removal, the method is less effective in wound debridement.[1,2] Clinicians must maintain the moisture level in the gauze to prevent dehydration and subsequent adherence to the wound bed, resulting in the wet-to-dry dressing. Clinicians should also monitor the periwound tissue for maceration.

Procedures

Similar to the wet-to-dry dressing, woven, sterile gauze with large pores is saturated with normal saline or potable tap water and then squeezed to damp.[16,19] The gauze is placed over the entire wound bed, covered, and allowed to remain for minutes to hours. The gauze is removed before complete drying and adherence to the wound bed.

Hydrotherapy

Whirlpool baths and soaks use potable tap water to soften, loosen, and remove adherent devitalized tissue and debris; hydrate the wound bed; and dilute the bacterial content of the wound.[2,5,17] Hydrotherapy is one of the oldest and most commonly used debridement methods.[2,17]

Indications

Hydrotherapy can be used on wounds with loosely adherent necrotic tissue, eschar, debris, and infected wounds.[2,17] Hydrotherapy can be used with other debridement methods, such as conservative sharp or autolytic debridement, to remove necrotic tissue.[2]

Contraindications

Hydrotherapy is not recommended for acute skin trauma. Hydrotherapy is a nonselective debridement method and can damage clean, granulating wounds.[2] Clinicians cannot control the turbine agitation force, and high pressures directed at the wound can traumatize healthy tissue. Immersion of the body part in water can increase the risk of maceration of the wound bed and peri-wound tissue and cross-contamination from the whirlpool tub, container, or immersion fluid.[2,21] Hydrotherapy debridement is neither cost-effective nor time effective because draining, proper cleaning and disinfecting, and refilling the tub or container after each patient must strictly adhere to infection control policies and procedures.[2,17,21]

Procedures

The whirlpool tub or container is filled with potable tap water between 92.0°F and 96.0°F (33.3°C and 35.5°C).[2,3] The body part and wound are submerged in water for 5 to 20 minutes.[2,3,17] After immersion, the body part is dried with clean towels and the periwound tissue with sterile gauze. Irrigation or conservative sharp debridement can be performed before applying the dressing.

Chemical Debridement

Chemical debridement is the use of sodium hypochlorite, hydrogen peroxide, acetic acid, chlorhexidine gluconate, or povidone-iodine in water-based solutions; silver or honey; or chemical-impregnated dressings to remove necrotic tissue, foreign material, and microorganisms from the wound bed. Clinicians should review the patient's health history and status in the decision to use this technique to lessen the risk of adverse reactions to chemical solutions and dressings.

Indications

Chemical debridement is indicated for wounds with a high risk of infection or clinically infected wounds. The antiseptic chemicals and compounds may serve as an alternative to topical or systemic antimicrobials in reducing the bioburden of the wound.[2] With these wounds, the priority is perhaps prevention of the transition to infection rather than the promotion of healing.[6] Chemical debridement may be used alone or with systemic antimicrobials to prevent or control infection.[9] Chemicals can also be used with wet-to-dry debridement.[6]

Contraindications

Clinicians should not use chemical solutions and chemical-impregnated dressings with acute skin trauma and the presence of healthy granulation tissue.[2,9,22,23] The use of many chemicals in full or diluted concentrations is controversial and thought to be cytotoxic to granulation tissue.[23] Clinicians should consider the risks of possible tissue damage against bioburden reduction with chemical debridement.

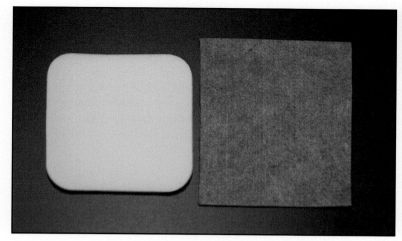

Figure 4-5. Silver-impregnated dressings. (Left) Foam. (Right) Alginate.

Procedures

Chemical solutions are applied directly to the wound bed through several methods. Woven, sterile gauze can be premoistened with solutions for wet-to-dry debridement. This technique is often used until the wound is debrided and cultured and antimicrobials are prescribed.[6] The use of chemical-impregnated dressings should follow the manufacturer's guidelines for indications, contraindications, and wear duration (Figure 4-5). Clinicians should closely monitor the patient for the development or progression of infection and adverse reactions with chemical debridement.

SUMMARY OF EVIDENCE

Limited reviews and randomized controlled trials provide evidence for the efficacy of debridement interventions in managing acute skin trauma. Despite the lack of evidence, debridement is considered the standard of care in clinical practice.[2] In an evidence-based review, autolytic debridement produced faster rates of healing than plain and impregnated gauze dressings in the management of postoperative incisions.[24] Individual trials in the review showed no differences in the rates of healing among the occlusive alginate, foam, and hydrocolloid dressings.[24] A separate evidence-based review examining diabetic foot ulcers demonstrated faster rates of healing with autolytic debridement compared with gauze dressings and conventional wound care.[25] The efficacy of chemical debridement interventions among uninfected[26] and contaminated and infected[27,28] acute and chronic wounds has been investigated in several reviews. The authors reported insufficient evidence to support silver-impregnated nonocclusive and occlusive dressings to prevent or manage infection. The authors of an evidence-based review examining healing of infected postoperative incisions found that honey and gauze dressings produced faster rates of healing compared with povidone-iodine and gauze dressings.[29] In a separate review comparing various techniques on the rates of debridement among infected postoperative incisions, the authors found no clear evidence for the most effective technique to create a clean wound bed.[30]

SUMMARY

Debridement, performed after cleansing, is the removal of necrotic tissue, foreign material, and microorganisms from the wound bed to create an optimal environment for healing. Debridement is necessary with some acute wounds to decrease the bacterial bioburden, enhance the body's defense mechanisms to lessen the risk of infection, create a viable wound bed for dressing application, and provide an unobstructed wound surface for the growth of new tissue and the progression of healing. Clinical decisions to determine whether debridement is warranted and which technique is appropriate are based on the patient's health status, wound characteristics, clinician knowledge and experience with the techniques, and applicable state practice acts. Debridement techniques available to clinicians include autolytic, conservative sharp, irrigation, scrubbing, wet to dry, wet to moist, hydrotherapy, and chemical. The techniques can be used alone or in combination with other methods to achieve healing outcomes. Several of these techniques can damage clean, granulating wounds; clinicians should carefully consider the risks of damage against the benefit of the technique before implementation.

REFERENCES

1. Attinger CE, Bulan EJ. Debridement. The key initial first step in wound healing. *Foot Ankle Clin.* 2001;6:627-660.

2. Albaugh K, Loehne H. Wound bed preparation/débridement. In: McCulloch JM, Kloth LC, eds. *Wound Healing: Evidence-Based Management.* 4th ed. F.A. Davis; 2010:155-179.

3. Ayello EA, Cuddigan J, Kerstein MD. Skip the knife: Debriding wounds without surgery. *Nursing.* 2002;32(9):58-63.

4. Myers BA. *Wound Management: Principles and Practice.* 2nd ed. Pearson Prentice Hall; 2008:70-93.

5. Beam JW, Buckley B, Holcomb WR, Ciocca M. National Athletic Trainers' Association position statement: Management of acute skin trauma. *J Athl Train.* 2016;51(12):1053-1070.

6. Ayello EA, Cuddigan JE. Debridement: Controlling the necrotic/cellular burden. *Adv Skin Wound Care.* 2004;17(2):66-75.

7. Honsik KA, Romeo MW, Hawley CJ, Romeo SJ, Romeo JP. Sideline skin and wound care for acute injuries. *Curr Sports Med Rep.* 2007;6(3):147-154.

8. Miller MG, Berry DC. Recognition and management of soft tissue injuries. In: Miller MG, Berry DC, eds. *Emergency Response Management for Athletic Trainers.* Wolters Kluwer/Lippincott Williams and Wilkins; 2010:283-309.

9. Gwynne B, Newton M. An overview of the common methods of wound debridement. *Br J Nurs.* 2006;15(19):S4-S10.

10. Alvarez O. Moist environment for healing: Matching the dressing to the wound. *Ostomy Wound Manage.* 1988;21:64-83.

11. Myers BA. *Wound Management: Principles and Practice.* 2nd ed. Pearson Prentice Hall; 2008:123-159.

12. Kannon GA, Garrett AB. Moist wound healing with occlusive dressings: A clinical review. *Dermatol Surg.* 1995;21(7):583-590.

13. Vowden KR, Vowden P. Wound debridement, part 2: Sharp techniques. *J Wound Care.* 1999;8(6):291-294.

14. Vowden K, Vowden P. Wound bed preparation. World Wide Wounds. 2002. Accessed May 3, 2022. http://www.worldwidewounds.com/2002/april/Vowden/Wound-Bed-Preparation.html

15. Calianno C, Jakubek P. Wound bed preperation: Laying the foundation for treating chronic wounds, part I. *Nursing.* 2006;36(2):70-71.

16. Hess CT. When to use gauze dressings. *Adv Skin Wound Care.* 2000;13(6):266-268.

17. Myers BA. *Wound Management: Principles and Practice.* 2nd ed. Pearson Prentice Hall; 2008:160-195.

18. Green VA, Carlson HC, Briggs RL, Stewart JL. A comparison of the efficacy of pulsed mechanical lavage with that of rubber-bulb syringe irrigation in removal of debris from avulsive wounds. *Oral Surg Oral Med Oral Pathol.* 1971;32(1):158-164.

19. Bradley M, Cullum N, Sheldon T. The debridement of chronic wounds: A systematic review. *Health Technol Assess.* 1999;3(17):1-78.

20. Singhal A, Reis ED, Kerstein MD. Options for nonsurgical debridement of necrotic wounds. *Adv Skin Wound Care.* 2001;14(2):96-100.

21. Hess CL, Howard MA, Attinger CE. A review of mechanical adjuncts in wound healing: Hydrotherapy, ultrasound, negative pressure therapy, hyperbaric oxygen, and electrostimulation. *Ann Plast Surg.* 2003;51(2):210-218.

22. Beam JW. Topical silver for infected wounds. *J Athl Train.* 2009;44(5):531-533.

23. O'Toole EA, Goel M, Woodley DT. Hydrogen peroxide inhibits human keratinocyte migration. *Dermatolog Surg.* 1996;22(6):525-529.

24. Lewis R, Whiting P, ter Riet G, O'Meara S, Glanville J. A rapid and systematic review of the clinical effectiveness and cost-effectiveness of debriding agents in treating surgical wounds healing by secondary intention. *Health Technol Assess.* 2001;5(14):1-131.

25. Elraiyah T, Domecq JP, Prutsky G, et al. A systematic review and meta-analysis of débridement methods for chronic diabetic foot ulcers. *J Vasc Surg.* 2016;63(2 suppl):37S-45S.

26. Storm-Versloot MN, Vos CG, Ubbink DT, Vermeulen H. Topical silver for preventing wound infection. *Cochrane Database Syst Rev.* 2010;3:CD006478.

27. Vermeulen H, van Hattem JM, Storm-Versloot MN, Ubbink DT, Westerbos SJ. Topical silver for treating infected wounds. *Cochrane Database Syst Rev.* 2007;1:CD005486.

28. Bergin S, Wraight P. Silver based wound dressings and topical agents for treating diabetic foot ulcers. *Cochrane Database Syst Rev.* 2006;1:CD005082.

29. Jull AB, Cullum N, Dumville JC, Westby MJ, Deshpande S, Walker N. Honey as a topical treatment for wounds. *Cochrane Database Syst Rev.* 2015;3:CD005083.

30. Smith F, Dryburgh N, Donaldson J, Mitchell M. Debridement for surgical wounds. *Cochrane Database Syst Rev.* 2013;9:CD006214.

5

DRESSINGS

Dressings for the management of acute skin trauma vary greatly in their materials, construction, and purposes. Dressing is the application of materials to cover the wound bed. The selection of an appropriate dressing is based on several factors, including patient and wound history and characteristics and the available dressing materials. Overall goals for dressings are to support and promote healing, prevent contamination and infection, and provide mechanical protection to the wound. This chapter begins with an overview of wound dressings commonly used in the management of acute skin trauma. The concept of a moist wound environment and its effects on healing are presented next. This is followed by a discussion on dressing functions, purposes, and goals and categories of dressings for acute wounds. The chapter concludes with guidelines and factors to consider for dressing selection and application.

WOUND DRESSINGS

Dressing of wounds has been practiced for centuries with a myriad of natural and synthetic materials and products. Currently, many advanced dressings are available made from a variety of materials. It has been estimated that more than 1000 dressing products are available to clinicians for

DOI: 10.1201/9781003523055-5

wound management.[1,2] Advancements in dressing construction, composition, and function over the last 60 years have changed the role of dressings in wound healing. Early dressings were used to cover the wound bed and often allowed for and were used to promote evaporative moisture loss and desiccation of the wound bed.[3] Drying of the wound bed and the formation of eschar (scab), with or without dressing use, were believed to promote healing and lessen the risk of infection. As a result, dressings designed to support desiccation of the wound bed became the standard of care. This standard underwent a drastic change as investigators revealed the importance of creating a moist environment for wound healing through occlusion of the wound.

MOIST WOUND HEALING

Work in the 1960s demonstrated faster rates of healing in occluded, moist wounds compared to air-exposed wounds in animal[4] and human[5] models. The action of trapping and balancing moisture next to the wound bed and preventing evaporative moisture loss produces a moist wound environment. Occlusion of the wound affects numerous host mechanisms to promote an environment beneficial to healing. The most important of these is perhaps the creation of a moist wound environment.[6] Management of exudate is conducted by moisture vapor transmission, the evaporation of fluid from the wound bed through the dressing. Moisture vapor transmission rate (MVTR) measures the speed at which fluid evaporates through a dressing in a given time[7] and is categorized as low (averaging 11 to 13 $g/m^2/h$), medium (averaging 33 $g/m^2/h$), and high (averaging 67 $g/m^2/h$).[8] An operational definition of moist wound healing for most partial- and full-thickness wounds is a dressing with low MVTR (< 30 $g/m^2/h$).[8] Although the exact moisture balance required in the wound bed to create the optimal moist environment is unknown,[9] low MVTR dressings (eg, films and hydrocolloids) have demonstrated faster rates of healing compared to medium (eg, foams and hydrogels) and high (eg, gauze) MVTR dressings among acute and chronic wounds.[8]

Although not fully understood, occlusion and a moist wound environment alter the microenvironment of the wound to facilitate vascular, cellular, and defense mechanisms during the healing process. A moist environment decreases the inflammatory phase[10] and prevents desiccation and the formation of eschar.[9] Fluid trapped over the wound contains enzymes that support autolytic debridement.[11-15] Occlusion and moist healing promote fibrinolysis to remove necrotic tissue and stimulate angiogenesis and the secretion of growth factors.[16] Phagocytic and lysosomal activity is enhanced with the presence of polymorphonuclear leukocytes, macrophages, lymphocytes, and monocytes.[17-20] Polymorphonuclear leukocytes infiltrate a moist wound more rapidly than a desiccated wound and have been shown to be bactericidal.[19-21] A moist, barrier-free wound bed allows activities in the proliferation phase to proceed unimpeded. Moist wound healing stimulates the production of platelet-derived, fibroblast, and epidermal growth factors in wound fluid.[16,22-26] The moist environment promotes an increase in fibroblast and keratinocyte proliferation and migration,[4,10,22,23,27,28] collagen synthesis,[29-32] endothelial cell growth,[23] angiogenesis,[16,33] and re-epithelization.[4,5,28-30,34-36] Moist wound healing continued through the maturation/remodeling phase may also produce improved cosmetic outcomes.[31,37-39] Occlusion of the wound bed and moist wound healing are created using moisture-retentive dressings, moist wound dressings, or occlusive dressings.

DRESSING FUNCTIONS

Acute wounds should be covered with a dressing to support healing rather than left uncovered and exposed to the external environment.[4,5,29,40-42] The purposes of a dressing are to complete healing in the shortest possible amount of time, prevent cross-contamination and infection, reduce pain, control and maintain moisture, and protect the wound from further trauma.[43,44] Each dressing has specific functions and is designed to be used individually or in combination with other dressings.

Dressings should maintain high humidity between the wound bed and dressing to create a moist environment to promote healing.[45-47] Wound dressings should manage and remove excess exudate to rid the wound bed of **exotoxins** and cell debris that can slow healing. The removal of excess exudate will also lower the risk of maceration.[45,48] Dressings should allow for gaseous exchange. Permeability to water vapor, oxygen, and carbon dioxide can assist the biochemical and cellular activity of the healing process.[45] Wound dressings should provide thermal insulation to the wound bed. A wound temperature at or near body temperature (98.6°F [37°C]) promotes an optimum healing rate.[45] Minimal exposure of the wound during dressing changes is also recommended to prevent temperature decreases.[45] The selection of dressings that can remain over the wound bed for longer periods of time will also lessen temperature changes. Dressings should be impermeable to microorganisms to prevent infection.[45] Wound dressings should be free of particles, fibers, and toxic contaminants that can produce scarring and encourage infection.[45] Dressings should also allow for dressing changes without additional trauma.[45] The adherence of a dressing to the wound surface from drying exudate can cause damage upon removal. Newly formed tissue can be stripped away, placing the wound back into the inflammatory healing phase.[45] An ideal dressing should also be sterile, nontoxic, and nonallergic with absorptive capabilities and a nonadherent surface. Additionally, the dressing should be physically strong in dry and wet conditions, able to remain on the wound surface for several days, easily disposed of, and cost-effective.[45,49]

DRESSING TYPES

Dressings used in the management of acute skin trauma can be categorized according to the material they are constructed from and their purpose, structure, and composition. Some dressings are designed to be used for a specific purpose, such as tissue approximation. Other dressings absorb and manage varying levels of exudate and can be used with several wound types. Primary dressings are applied directly on the wound bed, and secondary dressings are used in combination with primary dressings. The selection of an appropriate dressing can be confusing for clinicians based on the variety of choices and brands available. Successful management of acute skin trauma requires clinicians to understand wound etiology and types and know the construction and properties of common dressings. Our discussion includes the types, descriptions, indications, and contraindications for the dressing categories of nonocclusive and occlusive dressings.

Nonocclusive

Nonocclusive dressings are found in most athletic training facilities and are commonly used by clinicians for acute wounds. Nonocclusive dressings include woven, nonwoven, and impregnated sterile gauze; nonadherent pads; adhesive strips and patches; and wound closure strips. Table 5-1 contains information on nonocclusive dressings.

Table 5-1. Sample Nonocclusive Dressings[a]

Type	Manufacturer/Brand Name
Woven and nonwoven sterile gauze	Covidien Curity pads Johnson & Johnson gauze pads
Impregnated sterile gauze	Covidien Curity packing strip CURAD packing strip
Nonadherent pads	Covidien Telfa CURAD nonadherent pad
Adhesive strips and patches	Beiersdorf Coverlet Johnson & Johnson BAND-AID
Wound closure strips	3M Steri-Strip Smith & Nephew Leukostrip

[a]An alphabetical list of products. No endorsement is implied.

Woven, Nonwoven, and Impregnated Sterile Gauze; Nonadherent Pads; and Adhesive Strips and Patches

Woven, nonwoven, and impregnated sterile gauze is available in squares, rolls, packing strips, and sheets of varying sizes and shapes (Figure 5-1). Woven gauze is constructed from cotton yarn or thread woven into a fabriclike form.[9] Nonwoven gauze consists of polyester, rayon, or blends of fibers pressed together.[9] Each is available in various thicknesses or layers that correspond with the dressing ply. A 16-ply dressing has more layers and thickness than an 8-ply dressing, providing greater absorbency and padding. Woven gauze has an open or loose weave pattern compared to the closed or tight weave of nonwoven gauze. This closed pattern allows nonwoven gauze to absorb greater amounts of exudate from a wound. Impregnated gauze is woven gauze with compounds such as petrolatum, zinc, iodoform, or antimicrobials incorporated into the dressing.[9]

Nonadherent pads and adhesive strips and patches are available in a variety of sizes and shapes (Figure 5-2). Nonadherent pads are constructed of bonded inner, contact, and outer layers of cotton materials. The outer layers are polymer coated to provide a nonadherent surface upon contact with the wound bed. Some designs are impregnated with antimicrobials. Other designs are available with a nonadherent pad as the primary dressing incorporated into a nonocclusive fabric or occlusive film secondary dressing. These designs are referred to as island dressings (Figure 5-3). Adhesive strips and patches are manufactured with a multilayer cotton pad, often polymer coated, incorporated into a woven fabric or latex adhesive strip or patch. Some strips and patches are waterproof or impregnated with antimicrobials.

Indications

Woven and nonwoven gauze can be used as primary and secondary dressings with all uninfected and infected acute skin trauma.[9,50] When used as primary dressings, woven and nonwoven gauze should be applied in combination with topical antimicrobial agents[9,50] or premoistened with normal saline[51,52] or tap water to promote a moist wound environment. Gauze premoistened with normal saline or tap water can be used as a temporary primary dressing with all wounds to return an athlete or patient to activity immediately. Woven and nonwoven gauze are also effective on irregular body surfaces when other dressings will not adhere.[53] Anecdotally, the frequent dressing changes conducted with infected wounds allow gauze to be cost-effective compared with other dressings.[9]

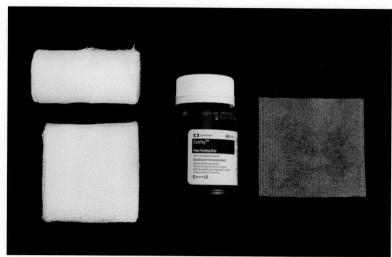

Figure 5-1. Woven, nonwoven, and impregnated sterile gauze. (Left) Gauze roll and squares. (Middle) Packing strips. (Right) Impregnated sheet.

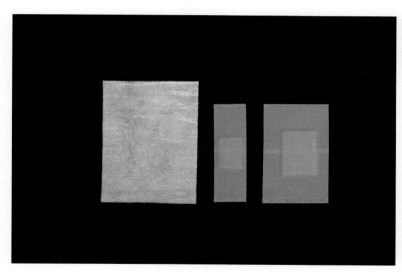

Figure 5-2. Nonadherent pads and adhesive strips and patches. (Left) Pad. (Middle) Strip. (Right) Patch.

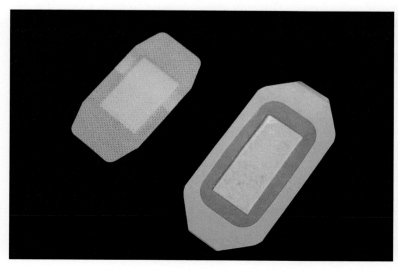

Figure 5-3. Island dressings. (Left) Nonadherent pad incorporated into secondary fabric dressing. (Right) Nonadherent pad incorporated into secondary film dressing.

Figure 5-4. Strike-through of a nonadherent pad.

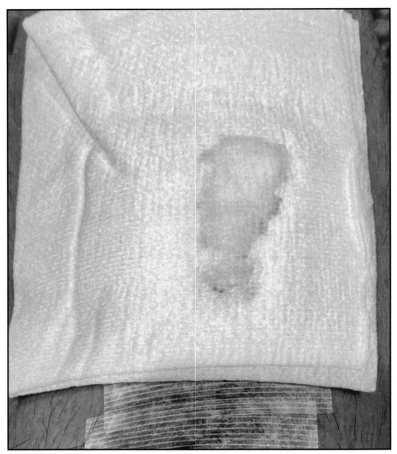

Woven, open weave gauze can be used with wet-to-moist debridement.[9,54,55] Woven, nonwoven, and impregnated gauze rolls and strips can be used to eliminate or pack dead space, prevent the closure of the wound surface, and allow healing from the base upward with puncture wounds with cavities.[7,51,56-58] Woven and nonwoven gauze used as a primary dressing requires daily dressing changes. As a secondary dressing, woven and nonwoven gauze can be applied over other nonocclusive and occlusive dressings to absorb excess exudate with heavily draining wounds. Heavy amounts of exudate can result in leakage and **strike-through** in the primary dressing (Figure 5-4). The accumulation of excessive exudate that leads to dressing saturation, leakage, or strike-through indicates the need for a dressing change. Gauze can also be used with primary dressings to provide additional padding and protection for the wound.

Nonadherent pads and adhesive strips and patches may be used as primary and secondary dressings with all uninfected and infected acute wounds.[9,50] Like gauze, nonadherent pads and adhesive strips and patches can be applied with topical antimicrobials or premoistened with normal saline or potable tap water and used as temporary primary dressings.[51,52] If applied without antimicrobials or premoistened, these dressings should only be used with superficial-thickness wounds with minimal exudate. Nonadherent pads and adhesive strips and patches can also be used on irregular body surfaces. Daily changes of nonadherent pads and adhesive strips and patches used as primary dressings are required. Nonadherent pads used as secondary dressings can provide additional padding to protect the wound. Adhesive strips and patches can assist in securing primary dressings to the periwound tissue.[53]

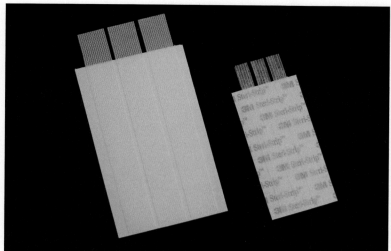

Figure 5-5. Wound closure strips.

Contraindications

Woven, nonwoven, and impregnated gauze; nonadherent pads; and adhesive strips and patches possess high permeability and can dry and adhere to the wound bed. Removal can result in trauma to the healing tissues. Clinicians should moisten the gauze, pads, strips, and patches through normal saline or tap water irrigation to rehydrate the dressings before removal.[9] The use of a topical anti-microbial with the dressings can lessen the risk of dressing desiccation and adherence to the wound and infection. Woven gauze can shed and leave fibers or lint in the wound bed upon removal. As a result, nonwoven gauze is better suited as a primary dressing. Impregnated gauze assists in maintaining a moist environment and does not adhere to the wound bed. These dressings do not absorb exudate but rather wick fluid away to a secondary dressing. Based on the impregnated chemical or compound, clinicians should carefully monitor the patient for the potential development of adverse reactions. Nonadherent pads and adhesive strips and patches have low absorbent properties, and the use of these dressings with draining wounds can result in maceration of the periwound tissue. Secondary gauze dressings should be changed daily with evidence of leakage, strike-through, or saturation with the exudate to prevent maceration.

Wound Closure Strips

Wound closure strips are constructed from nonwoven rayon/polyester/nylon filaments coated with a hypoallergenic adhesive material (Figure 5-5). Some strips contain an elastic material that allows for slight movement of the wound area while maintaining tissue approximation. Strips are available in various widths and lengths to accommodate different wound sizes and locations. The strips are packaged on a paper card and applied individually or together directly from the card.

Indications

Wound closure strips can be used as a primary dressing with uninfected traumatic lacerations and incisions and postoperative incisions with minimal static and dynamic tension that require tissue approximation.[59-61] Strips can also be used with sutures and staples to secure the wound edges. After the removal of sutures and staples, wound closure strips are commonly used for tissue approximation until the wound is healed. Wound closure strips can remain in place for 5 to 10 days or until the strips separate from the periwound tissue. Detailed instructions for the application of wound closure strips are found in the Application Guidelines section (see p.85).

Table 5-2. Sample Occlusive Dressings[a]	
Type	**Manufacturer/Brand Name**
Alginate	3M Tegaderm Alginate
	Covidien Curasorb
	Smith & Nephew ALGISITE M
Film	3M Tegaderm Transparent Film
	Johnson & Johnson Bioclusive Plus
	Kendall Transparent Film
Foam	3M Tegaderm Foam
	Kendall Foam
	Ferris PolyMem
Hydrogel	Covidien Aquaflo
	Spenco Aquaheal
Hydrocolloid	3M Tegaderm Hydrocolloid
	ConvaTec DuoDerm
Dermal adhesive	Ethicon Dermabond
	TissueSeal Histoacryl

[a]An alphabetical list of products. No endorsement is implied.

Contraindications

Wound closure strips should not be used for the closure of infected lacerations and incisions. Strips are inappropriate for wounds under high tension that do not allow for simple, manual approximation of the wound edges. Wound closure strips will not adhere to wet and oily skin or hairy body areas. The skin should be clean and dry for application. Clinicians can enhance the adherence of the strips with the application of tincture of benzoin on the periwound tissue.

Occlusive

Semipermeable and impermeable occlusive dressings promote a moist wound environment to facilitate healing and reduce the risk of infection. Many designs of occlusive dressings are available to the clinician. This discussion focuses on alginates, films, foams, hydrogels, hydrocolloids, and dermal adhesives for the management of acute skin trauma. Table 5-2 lists information on occlusive dressings.

Alginates

Calcium alginate dressings are derived from specific types of brown seaweed and are converted into woven or nonwoven fiber sheets, pads, or ropes in various sizes (Figure 5-6). Sheets are appropriate for acute skin trauma. When the dressing is applied to a wound, an ion exchange between the dressing fibers and wound exudate produces a hydrophilic gel that creates and maintains a moist wound environment. This gel prevents the dressing from adhering to the wound bed. The permeable dressings can absorb and remove significant amounts of exudate within the wound. Clinicians can cut alginate sheets to the size and shape of the wound. Alginates do not allow for visual inspection of

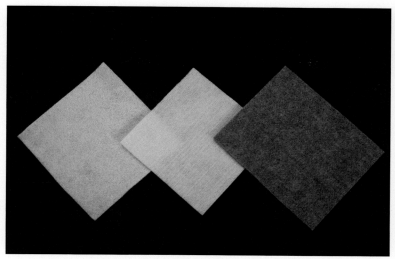

Figure 5-6. Alginate dressings. (Left and middle) Sheet dressings. (Right) Silver-impregnated sheet dressing.

the wound bed while in place. Most sheet alginates are nonadhesive and require a secondary dressing. Some alginate dressings are available with impregnated silver for antimicrobial purposes and others with alginate-honey or alginate-hydrocolloid combinations in sheet forms.

Indications

Alginates can be used as primary dressings with partial- to full-thickness abrasions, avulsions, blisters, and lacerations and incisions with adequate tissue approximation.[9,62,63] Alginates can effectively manage the moderate to heavy exudate that accompanies partial- to full-thickness wounds. The dressings can remain on the wound bed for up to 7 days in the absence of dressing integrity issues or clinical features of infection or adverse reactions.[6] Based on the high absorbency properties of the dressing, alginates can be used with infected wounds to manage the significant amounts of exudate typically produced by infection.[7,9,64] Daily dressing changes are required with infected wounds.

Contraindications

Alginates are not appropriate for use with minimally draining wounds. The high absorbency can desiccate the wound bed and allow the dressing to adhere to the wound. Removal of the dressing can cause further trauma to the wound bed. Remoistening the dressing with normal saline or potable tap water irrigation before removal is warranted. The hydrophilic gel produced by alginates can have a foul odor among some patients. Clinicians should be careful and not mistake the odor for the development of infection.[6,9] The selection of an appropriate secondary dressing is necessary to adhere alginates to the periwound tissue, support the creation of a moist environment, and provide occlusion for the wound.

Films

Film dressings are thin, transparent sheets of polyurethane with an adhesive backing on one side (Figure 5-7). The dressings are water vapor, oxygen, and carbon dioxide permeable and microorganism and liquid impermeable. Film dressings are available in various widths and lengths to cover a variety of wound sizes. The dressings are flexible and can adhere to most body areas and contours. Trimming or cutting the dressing can be difficult because of the adhesive backing and

Figure 5-7. Film dressings.

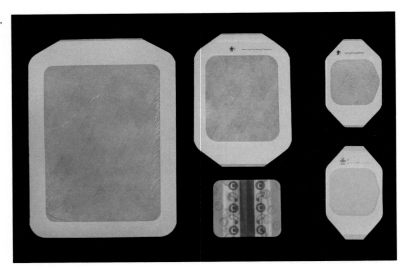

Figure 5-8. Film dressing over a wound.

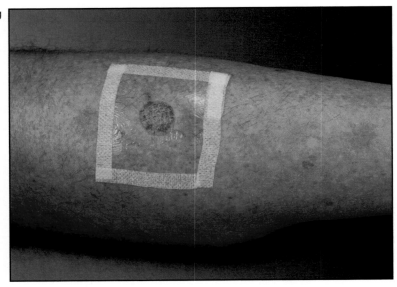

flexible construction and can affect the application sequence. Film dressings are nonabsorbent but trap fluid over the wound bed to create a moist environment. The moisture prevents the adhesive dressing from adhering to the wound bed. The thin, transparent design of the films allows for visual inspection of the wound without removing the dressing (Figure 5-8). However, the trapping of exudate and fluids over the wound will obstruct the view of the wound bed. Film dressings are waterproof and allow the patient to bathe and shower.

Indications

Films should be used as primary dressings with superficial- to partial-thickness abrasions, avulsions, blisters, incisions, lacerations, and punctures with low levels of exudate.[9,40,42,44,65,66] Films can remain over the wound bed for up to 3 to 7 days without dressing integrity problems or clinical features of infection or adverse reactions.[6,7,9,67,68] Film dressings are not appropriate as primary dressings with infected wounds. Films can be difficult to apply because of their thin, flexible construction.

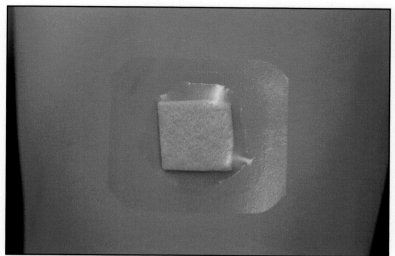

Figure 5-9. Secondary film dressing with a primary alginate dressing on a wound model.

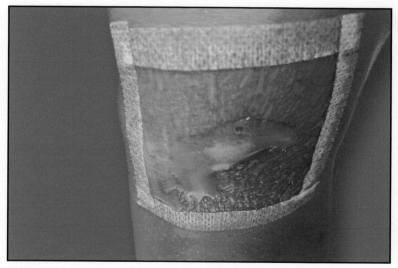

Figure 5-10. Channels in a film dressing.

Films can be used as secondary dressings with superficial- to full-thickness wounds. They can be used with alginates, foams, and hydrogels to secure these dressings and provide occlusion (Figure 5-9).[67] In combination with other occlusive dressings, films provide additional adherence for the primary dressing to the periwound tissue and prevent leakage of excess exudate from heavily draining wounds.[53] They can also be applied over lacerations and traumatic and postoperative incisions that are closed with sutures,[59,69-73] staples,[69] or dermal adhesives.[59,69]

Contraindications

Film dressings should not be used as primary dressings on wounds with moderate to heavy levels of exudate. Excessive fluid can accumulate under the dressing and lead to the development of **channels** in the dressing (Figure 5-10). These channels can lift the perimeter of the dressing from the periwound tissue and result in leakage, compromising the occlusive barrier properties, promoting desiccation, and increasing the risk of contamination and infection.[9,41,53,74,75] A dressing change or reassessment of dressing selection is needed with excessive accumulation of fluid

Figure 5-11. Fluid visible under a film dressing.

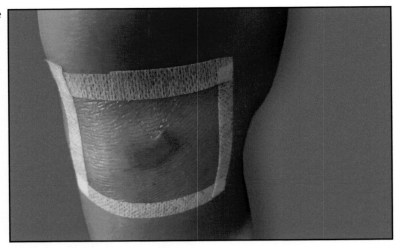

Figure 5-12. Foam dressings. (Right and left) Non-adhesive foams. (Middle) Foams incorporated into secondary film dressings.

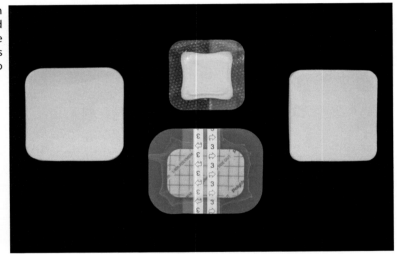

or leakage. Desiccation and adherence of the dressing over the wound bed require irrigation with normal saline or potable tap water before removal to prevent damage to the healing tissues.[9] The collection of fluid under the transparent film dressing will have a brownish color (Figure 5-11). Clinicians should not confuse this fluid with infection.[13] The thin construction of films produces minimal insulation to the wound. Clinicians should only apply the dressings to intact, dry skin to ensure adhesion to the periwound tissue. Monitor the removal of film dressings because the adhesive backing can damage the periwound tissue.

Foams

Foams are semipermeable dressings with a hydrophilic inner layer of polyurethane foam and a hydrophobic outer membrane of polyester, silicone, or Gore-Tex (W. L. Gore & Associates; Figure 5-12).[6,76,77] Foams are permeable to gases and water. The dressings possess a moderate to high MVTR and high absorbency, allowing them to manage heavy amounts of exudate.[8] Foams create a moist wound environment and provide insulation and protection to the wound. Like other occlusive dressings, the moist environment prevents the foam from adhering to the wound bed. Foams vary

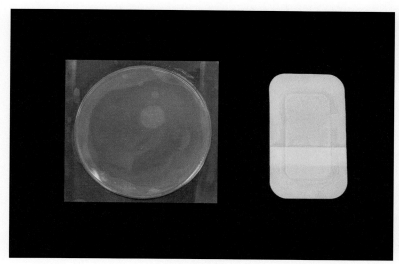

Figure 5-13. Hydrogel dressings. (Left) Sheet dressing. (Right) Hydrogel incorporated into secondary film dressing.

in size and thickness based on the manufacturer and are available with adhesive or nonadhesive borders. Foams with a nonadhesive border require a secondary dressing, such as a film. Some foams are incorporated into a secondary film dressing, allowing bathing and showering. The film backing can affect the MVTR of the dressing.[9] Clinicians can cut the dressings to fit the shape of the wound. Several designs are impregnated with different concentrations and release rates of silver.

Indications

Foams can be used as primary dressings on partial- to full-thickness wounds with moderate to heavy exudate, such as abrasions, avulsions, blisters, and lacerations and incisions with adequate tissue approximation.[9,62,63] Foam dressings can remain over the wound bed for up to 3 to 7 days.[6,7,9,67,68] During this period, dressing changes are required with excessive accumulation of exudate and dressing saturation, leakage, or clinical features of infection or adverse reactions.[7,9,41] Foams can be used for contaminated and clinically infected wounds but require daily changes.[7,9,64,78]

Contraindications

Foam dressings are not indicated for superficial-thickness, minimally draining, or dry wounds. Their high MVTR and absorbency can further desiccate the wound bed. If allowed to dry while over the wound, foams can adhere to the wound bed. Irrigation should be used to moisten the dressing before removal. The secondary dressing used with nonadhesive foams should promote a moist wound environment, support occlusion of the wound, and secure the foam dressing to the periwound tissue.

Hydrogels

Hydrogel dressings are a network of hydrophilic polymer chains consisting of 80% to 99% water and are available in 3-dimensional sheets or amorphous gels (Figure 5-13).[49,76] Hydrogel sheets are used with acute skin trauma. The dressings are permeable to gases and water vapor, and permeability to microorganisms is influenced by the type of secondary dressing used.[79] Sheet hydrogels are available in square or disc shapes and can be cut to fit the size of the wound. Most sheet hydrogels are nonadhesive and require a secondary dressing for adherence and occlusion. Some hydrogels are incorporated into a film secondary dressing and allow for bathing and showering. The dressings absorb minimal to moderate exudate amounts and create a moist wound environment. Based on their high water content, hydrogels can donate moisture to the wound bed, lessening the risk of desiccation in minimally draining superficial-thickness wounds.[80,81] They are semitransparent and allow for partial visual assessment of the wound bed. When initially applied, hydrogels have a cooling effect on the wound surface. They also protect the wound as a primary dressing based on their thickness and can be used in combination with other materials to lessen friction and shear forces.

Indications

Hydrogels can be used as primary dressings with superficial- to partial-thickness abrasions, avulsions, blisters, incisions, lacerations, and punctures with minimal to moderate levels of exudate.[6,9,13,40,42,44,51,80] Clinicians can also use them with dry wounds to remoisten the wound bed. Hydrogels should not be used with infected wounds. Hydrogels can remain over the wound bed for up to 1 to 7 days in the absence of dressing integrity issues or clinical features of infection and adverse reactions.[6,7,67]

Contraindications

Hydrogels are not appropriate for wounds with heavy exudate. Maceration of the wound bed and periwound tissue can result from excessive exudate; high water content; and slow, minimal absorption properties of hydrogels.[3,13] Water donation to the wound bed can dehydrate the dressing if left over the wound for an extended period. If the dressing desiccates and adheres to the wound, irrigation is needed for removal. Nonadhesive discs or square hydrogels require a secondary dressing for adherence to the periwound tissue and to provide occlusion. Because of their construction and thickness, hydrogels are heavier than other occlusive dressings. Therefore, they may not be the best choice for athletes based on the high levels of activity and movement, resultant perspiration, and potential failure of the secondary dressing to maintain adherence of the hydrogel to the periwound tissue. Hydrogels intended for use as primary dressings are available in single, sterile packages. Other hydrogel products in nonsterile packaging should not be applied directly over the wound bed as a primary dressing. These hydrogels are combined with primary and secondary dressings to lessen friction and shear forces.

Hydrocolloids

Hydrocolloid dressings consist of a waterproof outer polyurethane film or foam with an inner self-adhesive gel-forming mass containing particles of carboxymethyl cellulose, gelatin, and pectin (Figure 5-14).[6,82] The dressings are impermeable to gases, water vapor, and microorganisms.[6] When applied to a wound, hydrocolloids interact with the exudate to form a cohesive or mobile gel, facilitating a moist wound environment, insulating the wound, and preventing dressing adherence to the wound bed and damage upon removal.[6,82] Hydrocolloids are wafer-type sheet dressings available in various sizes and thicknesses. The conformable dressings can be cut to fit the size and shape of the wound and do not require a secondary dressing. Hydrocolloids can manage minimal to moderate amounts of exudate and absorb fluids slowly. The opaque dressings do not allow visual inspection of the wound bed; patients can bathe and shower while the dressing is over the wound.

Indications

Hydrocolloids should be used as primary dressings on partial- to full-thickness abrasions, avulsions, blisters, and lacerations and traumatic and postoperative incisions with adequate tissue approximation with minimal to moderate exudate.[62,70-72,83] Trimming to round all corners of the dressing will prevent the edges from rolling with contact with clothing. Hydrocolloids can remain

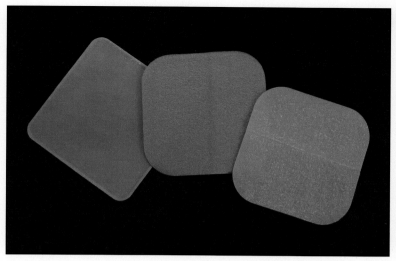

Figure 5-14. Hydrocolloid dressings.

over the wound bed for 5 to 7 days without leakage, separation of the dressing edges from the periwound tissue, bunching of the dressing, or clinical features of infection or adverse reactions.[6,7,67,68] The dressings are not appropriate for infected wounds. Hydrocolloids can be used as secondary dressings for lacerations and traumatic and postoperative incisions managed with sutures,[59,69,70-73] staples,[69] or dermal adhesives.[59,69]

Contraindications

Hydrocolloids should not be used as a primary dressing with superficial-thickness, dry wounds. The dressings are also inappropriate for heavily draining wounds because of their slow absorption properties. The adhesive backing of hydrocolloids can damage the periwound tissue upon removal. Irrigation with normal saline or tap water can assist in dressing removal if necessary. The gel created by hydrocolloids under the dressing can have a foul odor. This odor should not be mistaken for infection.[6,9] The gel will remain over the wound bed after removing the dressing. The gel can be left in place when applying a fresh occlusive dressing if there are no clinical signs of infection or adverse reactions. Inspection of the wound or transition to another dressing type will require the removal of the gel through irrigation. The absorption of exudate and the production of this gel will cause hydrocolloids to expand and swell over the wound bed (Figure 5-15). Direct force from contact with other individuals, equipment, or playing surfaces among athletes and active individuals can compromise the integrity of the dressing.[53] The contact can rupture the dressing or force exudate to the dressing perimeter, creating channels and possible leakage.[53]

Dermal Adhesives

Dermal adhesives are 2-octyl cyanoacrylate or n-butyl-2-cyanoacrylate sterile, liquid compounds (Figure 5-16). The adhesives are supplied in a single-use ampoule or pen applicator forms. The adhesives polymerize upon contact with tissues, forming a transparent occlusive dressing and tissue bond.[84,85] The polymerization is **exothermic** and produces a small amount of heat at the tissue site. Complete drying and bonding strength of the adhesive occurs within minutes or when the adhesive is no longer tacky.[84] After polymerization, a partial visual assessment of the wound can be conducted. Dermal adhesives allow for gentle bathing and showering, but patients should avoid soaking the site. Occlusive films and hydrocolloids[59,69] or nonocclusive gauze, nonadherent pads, or adhesive strips or patches[7,9,43,69] may be used as secondary dressings after complete polymerization.

Figure 5-15. Expansion and swelling of a hydrocolloid over the wound.

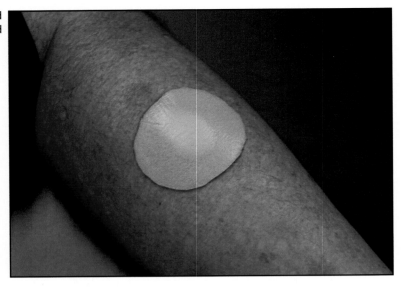

Figure 5-16. Dermal adhesives. (Left) Ampoule (Histoacryl® | H.B. Fuller). (Right) Pen applicator.

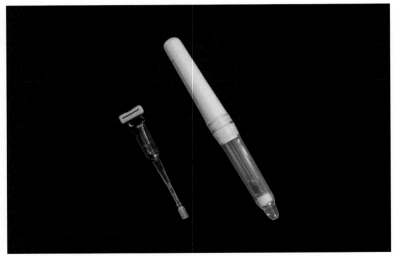

Indications

Dermal adhesives can be used as primary dressings with lacerations and traumatic and postoperative incisions in areas of low skin tension that require tissue approximation.[60,61,86,87] The topical adhesives can be applied with, but not replace, deep dermal sutures.[84,85] The adhesives normally remain over the wound and bond the tissue edges for 5 to 10 days and then begin to **slough off**.[84,85] Clinicians should monitor the patient and wound for clinical features of infection and adverse reactions during this period. Dermal adhesives should not be used for tissue approximation of infected wounds. The adhesive is delivered to dry, easily approximated wound edges. Detailed instructions for the application of dermal adhesives are provided in the Application Guidelines section (see p.85).

Contraindications

Dermal adhesives are used for topical application only and should not be applied under the skin. Underlying tissues will not absorb the adhesive, and a delay in wound healing, foreign body reaction, or adverse cosmetic outcomes can result.[84] Adhesives are inappropriate for wounds in areas of high skin tension and around joints. Clinicians should also avoid their use on **mucosal surfaces**, **mucocutaneous junctions**, and wounds subject to prolonged moisture. Dermal adhesives should only be applied to dry skin with minimal hair to ensure tissue approximation. Clinicians should exercise caution during application because the adhesive can bond to gloves and instruments. The application of excessive amounts of adhesive will increase heat production from the polymerization and can cause damage to the skin. The heavy pressure of the applicator tip on the wound edges during application can cause separation of the edges and loss of approximation. Topical antimicrobial creams or ointments applied over the adhesive can weaken the polymerization and result in wound dehiscence.[84]

SUMMARY OF EVIDENCE

Evidence-based medicine reviews and clinical investigations have focused on the efficacy of nonocclusive and occlusive dressings for healing and infection rates and pain levels among various wounds. An evidence-based review found occlusive dressings produced faster rates of healing compared with nonocclusive dressings among split-thickness skin graft (STSG) donor sites.[65] The STSG is equivalent to a superficial- to partial-thickness abrasion.[88] Hydrocolloid and film dressings were superior to nonocclusive dressings, and hydrocolloids were favored over other occlusive dressings for rates of healing. The authors of a separate evidence-based review examining STSG and postoperative incisions reported no differences in the rates of healing among nonocclusive and occlusive dressings.[66] Several reviews investigated the efficacy of nonocclusive and occlusive dressings impregnated with silver on uninfected[89] and contaminated and infected[78,90] acute and chronic wounds. The findings demonstrated no support for the use of silver-impregnated dressings to enhance the rates of healing. The efficacy of nonocclusive and occlusive dressings for the closure of traumatic and postoperative wounds has been examined in 2 reviews. One review examined standard wound closure (sutures, staples, and wound closure strips) and dermal adhesives among postoperative incisions and found sutures lessened the rates of dehiscence; wound closure strips improved surgeons' ratings of cosmetic appearance; and sutures, staples, and wound closure strips increased surgeons' satisfaction ratings for ease of use.[61] The authors revealed inconsistent findings for the time to complete closure between standard wound closure techniques and dermal adhesives.[61] Another review investigated the closure of traumatic lacerations with standard wound closure techniques (sutures, staples, and wound closure strips) and dermal adhesives.[60] The findings demonstrated dermal adhesives lowered levels of pain, the time to close the wound, and the rate of erythema. However, dermal adhesives increased the risk of dehiscence compared to standard wound closure techniques. The authors revealed no differences in cosmetic outcomes, and standard wound closure techniques were superior to dermal adhesives for ease of use.[60] Several small experimental and clinical investigations examining the rates of healing in standardized partial-thickness abrasions showed hydrocolloids and films were favored over nonocclusive dressings,[42] other occlusive dressings (foams and hydrogels),[40,44] and no dressing.[40,42] Authors examining the efficacy of hydrocolloids used as secondary dressings on the rates of healing for sutured and nonsutured lacerations and incisions revealed inconsistent findings compared with nonocclusive dressings.[37,70,91]

Several evidence-based reviews have examined the rates of infection among nonocclusive and occlusive dressings. One review revealed that occlusive dressings produced lower rates of infection compared with nonocclusive dressings among STSGs.[65] Another review of 75 studies (3047 acute and chronic wounds) compared nonocclusive and occlusive dressings and found overall infection rates of 2.6% and 7.1%, respectively.[92] The authors of an evidence-based review examining closure of postoperative incisions demonstrated no differences in the rates of infection between nonocclusive standard wound closure (sutures, staples, and wound closure strips) and occlusive dermal adhesives.[61] Several reviews have examined the efficacy of nonocclusive and occlusive dressings impregnated with silver on the rates of infection in uninfected[89] and contaminated and infected[78,90] acute and chronic wounds. The authors reported no clear evidence to support the use of silver-impregnated dressings to prevent or control infection. The efficacy of nonocclusive and occlusive dressings used as secondary dressings for postoperative incisions closed with sutures, staples, dermal adhesives, or a combination of these techniques on the rates of surgical site infection was examined in a review.[69] The findings demonstrated no clear evidence for differences in the rates of infection between nonocclusive and occlusive dressings and no dressing. The authors also reported no clear evidence for the most effective dressing to lessen the rates of surgical site infection among postoperative incisions.[69]

Levels of pain with the use of nonocclusive and occlusive dressings have been reported. One review found occlusive dressings used as primary dressings lowered greater levels of pain on visual analog scales at rest and with ambulation than nonocclusive dressings in the management of STSGs.[65] Several experimental and clinical investigations revealed decreased levels of pain with hydrocolloids used as secondary dressings compared with nonocclusive secondary dressings in the management of sutured lacerations and postoperative incisions.[37,93,94]

SELECTION AND APPLICATION

With an understanding of the basic categories of dressings and their properties and purposes, clinicians can select and apply a dressing to promote healing, lessen the risk of infection and adverse reactions, and protect the wound (Table 5-3). The selection of a dressing can be challenging because no one nonocclusive or occlusive dressing is appropriate for every wound.[45,95] Additionally, few dressings are suited for a single wound over the complete healing process.[43] The selection of an appropriate dressing is based on multiple factors; integrating these factors will guide the clinician in choosing the most effective dressing for the patient and wound.

Factors to Consider

Dressing selection is determined by several factors including characteristics of the wound; the types and availability of dressings; and the health, needs, and activity level of the patient. The selection process begins by identifying the primary goal or purpose of the dressing, which is normally complete healing in the shortest amount of time.[43,44] However, interim goals or priorities for the patient and wound during the healing sequence can become the most important to address. For example, the control of heavy exudate in a full-thickness abrasion must be managed to lessen the risk of maceration and dressing failure. Reducing friction and shear with a calcaneal blister is required to protect the wound from further trauma. The management of clinical infection or allergic contact dermatitis can alter goals and influence dressing selection. After identifying the dressing goal or purpose, clinicians can begin the selection process.

Table 5-3. Wound Dressing Summary

Dressing	Indications	Advantages	Disadvantages
Woven, nonwoven, and impregnated sterile gauze	• Superficial- to full-thickness abrasions, avulsions, blisters, lacerations, punctures, and traumatic and postoperative incisions • Wounds with low to heavy exudate levels	• High absorbency • Cost-effective with frequent changes • Readily available • Use on infected wounds • Provide protection of wound • Use as a secondary dressing • Use as a temporary dressing	• Require daily changes • High permeability • Can adhere to a dry wound bed • Can leave fibers/lint in wound bed • Require a secondary dressing • Lower rates of healing and higher rates of infection compared with occlusive dressings
Nonadherent pads and adhesive strips and patches	• Superficial- to full-thickness abrasions, avulsions, blisters, lacerations, punctures, and traumatic and postoperative incisions • Wounds with low to heavy exudate levels	• Readily available • Use on infected wounds • Use as a temporary dressing • Use as a secondary dressing	• Require daily changes • High permeability • Can adhere to a dry wound bed • Low absorptive properties • Require a secondary dressing (nonadherent pads) • Lower rates of healing and higher rates of infection compared with occlusive dressings
Wound closure strips	• Lacerations and traumatic and postoperative incisions with minimal static and dynamic tension requiring tissue approximation	• Use with and following removal of sutures and staples	• Not for use with infected wounds • Not for use with wounds under high tension • Can increase risk of dehiscence • Will not adhere to wet and oily skin or hairy body areas

continued

Table 5-3. Wound Dressing Summary (continued)

Dressing	Indications	Advantages	Disadvantages
Alginates	• Partial- to full-thickness abrasions, avulsions, blisters, and lacerations and incisions with adequate tissue approximation • Wounds with moderate to heavy exudate levels	• Promote autolytic debridement • High absorbency • Use on infected wounds with daily changes	• Do not allow visual inspection of wound bed • Most require a secondary dressing • Not for use on minimally draining wounds • Can adhere to a dry wound bed • Can produce a foul odor
Films	• Superficial- to partial-thickness abrasions, avulsions, blisters, incisions, lacerations, and punctures • Wounds with minimal exudate levels	• Promote autolytic debridement • Impermeable to microorganisms • Flexible and waterproof • Allow for visual inspection of wound bed • Use as a secondary dressing	• Nonabsorbent • Not for use with heavily draining wounds • Not for use with infected wounds • Can adhere to a dry wound bed • Can be difficult to apply • Adhesive can damage the periwound tissue upon removal • Do not insulate wound
Foams	• Partial- to full-thickness abrasions, avulsions, blisters, and lacerations and incisions with adequate tissue approximation • Wounds with moderate to heavy exudate levels	• Promote autolytic debridement • High absorbency • Use on infected wounds with daily changes • Insulate and protect wound bed	• Do not allow visual inspection of wound bed • Most require a secondary dressing • Not for use on minimally draining wounds • Can adhere to a dry wound bed

continued

Table 5-3. Wound Dressing Summary (continued)

Dressing	Indications	Advantages	Disadvantages
Hydrogels	• Superficial- to partial-thickness abrasions, avulsions, blisters, incisions, lacerations, and punctures • Wounds with minimal to moderate exudate levels	• Promote autolytic debridement • Can donate moisture to wound bed • Allow for partial visual inspection of wound bed • Protect wound bed • Use on dry wounds	• Most require a secondary dressing • Not for use with infected wounds • Not for use with heavily draining wounds • Can increase risk of maceration • Can dehydrate • Heavier than most dressings
Hydrocolloids	• Partial- to full-thickness abrasions, avulsions, blisters, and lacerations and traumatic and postoperative incisions with adequate tissue approximation • Wounds with minimal to moderate exudate levels	• Promote autolytic debridement • Do not require a secondary dressing • Waterproof • Insulate wound bed • Use as a secondary dressing • Impermeable to water vapor and microorganisms	• Slow absorption of exudate • Not for use with infected wounds • Do not allow visual inspection of wound bed • Not for use with dry or heavily draining wounds • Can damage the periwound tissue upon removal • Can leave gel residue on wound bed • Will expand/swell with and following athletic activity • Can be messy and produce foul odor
Dermal adhesives	• Lacerations and traumatic and postoperative incisions requiring tissue approximation in areas of low skin tension	• Allow for partial visual inspection of wound bed • Waterproof • May shorten closure time • Anesthetic not required	• Not for use with infected wounds • Not for use in areas of high skin tension, around joints, and on mucosal surfaces and mucocutaneous junctions • Should not be applied under the skin • Can increase risk of dehiscence

Wound

Characteristics of the wound including the type, depth of tissue damage, amount of exudate, condition of the wound and periwound tissue, phase of healing, mechanism of injury, location, amount of necrotic tissue, and presence of infection can influence the effectiveness of the dressing and the rate of healing. The wound type will determine the depth of tissue damage, amount of exudate, and condition of the periwound tissue. Deeper wounds, such as an open, full-thickness blister, will produce heavier amounts of exudate than a superficial-thickness laceration. A dressing with high absorbency properties is needed to manage large amounts of exudate. A superficial-thickness wound requires a less absorbent dressing or a moisture-donating dressing if the wound bed is dry. The condition of the wound edges and periwound tissue will determine the method of wound closure. Wound edges that can be approximated are closed by **primary closure** with wound closure strips, dermal adhesives, sutures, or staples. Wound edges that cannot be approximated are closed by **secondary closure** with nonocclusive or occlusive dressings. Wound healing is a balancing process between the wound and local and systematic environments with dynamic cellular and chemical activities.[3,43] Cellular and chemical activities diminish as healing progresses, resulting in decreased levels of exudate and new epithelial growth.[43] Dressing purposes and selection should correspond to the changing wound environment during the healing process. Based on the mechanism of injury, the wound and periwound tissue may require protection from shear and tensile forces and loads to limit further trauma. Wound location can reveal the amount of tension, shear, and friction applied to the body during ambulation and activity that can affect the dressing integrity, physical properties, and performance. Excessive shear and friction can lessen the ability of a dressing to adhere to the periwound tissue. An alternative dressing may be required to cover and protect the wound in this situation. Necrotic tissue or eschar within the wound from delayed inspection or inappropriate treatment can delay healing. Debridement is indicated for the removal of the tissue and debris to create an environment suitable for healing. Autolytic debridement with occlusive dressings, wet to moist using gauze, or conservative sharp with sterile instruments may be appropriate. Clinical infection of the wound requires the use of only those dressings indicated to lessen the risk of further complications. Clinicians can manage the heavy drainage produced by infection with sterile gauze, alginate, or foam dressings. Regardless of dressing choice, daily changes are required.

Dressing

Dressing options for the clinician are numerous. Factors such as absorbency, permeability, conformability to body area, mass/weight, ease of use and removal, and availability and cost should be used to determine the most effective dressing to promote healing.[43] Absorbency and permeability to fluid, gases, and microorganisms will influence the MVTR[7]; moisture balance in the wound bed[7-9]; and risk of maceration,[96] cross-contamination, and infection.[74,75,97] The selected dressing should create and maintain a moist, not wet, wound environment and be impermeable to bacteria while over the wound. A dressing that is too absorbent can desiccate the wound and delay healing. Conformability and mass will affect the ability of the dressing to maintain adherence to the periwound tissue during daily and athletic activities. Primary occlusive dressings with adhesive backing can remain over the wound for multiple days to promote an environment conducive to healing. The use of a secondary dressing can enhance conformability and adherence during practices and competitions for athletes. User-friendly application and removal will prevent additional trauma to the wound bed and increase patient compliance.[45] With experience, clinicians can apply dressings in a timely manner. The ability of occlusive dressings to remain over the wound bed for days will also lessen dressing changes and application time and increase patient compliance. Removal should be cautiously approached because dressings can adhere to the wound bed. The availability of dressing types often influences selection. Purchasing a wide selection of nonocclusive and occlusive dressings is likely not cost-effective for most athletic training facilities.[53] Clinicians may need to select and use an alternative dressing when products are not available. Dressing costs should also be considered.

Less expensive nonocclusive dressings such as gauze are appropriate for wounds requiring daily changes. Occlusive dressings should be used when the dressing can remain on the wound bed for several days.[9] Although more expensive per individual dressing, occlusive dressings require less frequent changes, resulting in less overall costs (eg, product and personnel costs). Based on the size of an occlusive dressing, clinicians may cut multiple dressings from the original sheet. For example, clinicians can cut multiple dressings based on wound size, shape, and location from a 15 cm × 15 cm hydrocolloid sheet. Store the remaining unused sheet in the original packaging and use it before the expiration date.

Patient

Patient factors are critical in the selection of a dressing intervention. Patient health status, allergies, activity (eg, sport or occupation), setting (eg, indoor, outdoor, or aquatics), and daily activities should be considered. Comorbidities such as diabetes[98] and malnutrition[99] may increase the risk of infection and contribute to a delay in healing. Topical or systematic steroids,[100,101] nonsteroidal anti-inflammatories,[102,103] and cyclooxygenase-2 inhibitors[104] commonly used by patients may negatively affect wound healing. Although these factors may impact normal wound healing, the influence on dressing selection is minimal.[43] However, clinicians should consider these factors in cases of delayed wound healing. Allergies to dressing materials used to treat acute skin trauma may eliminate certain types from the selection process. Polyurethane, gelatin, pectin, glycerin, and carboxymethyl cellulose are used to construct occlusive dressings and can lead to adverse reactions in susceptible patients. Work and sports equipment and settings can influence dressing integrity and compliance. Protective equipment (eg, shoes, boots, shin guards, and knee and elbow pads), uniforms, work and sports demands (eg, kneeling, sitting, and sliding), and environmental conditions (eg, heat, humidity, and rain) can loosen or dislodge the dressing. Separation of the dressing edges from the periwound tissue resulting in the leakage of exudate or complete removal of the dressing can compromise the barrier properties and increase the risk of cross-contamination and infection and lead to desiccation of the wound.[41,74,75] Frequent integrity issues can lead to additional dressing changes, impacting costs and patient compliance. Daily activities and therapeutic interventions can also affect dressing integrity and effectiveness. Bathing and showering should only be conducted with those dressings allowed by the manufacturer for such use. Films and hydrocolloids and foams and hydrogels with a film secondary dressing allow patients to bathe and shower. Patients may require alternative therapeutic interventions to lessen the risk of direct contact with the modalities with the dressing. The use of aquatic activities (eg, whirlpool and pool) while the wound is healing may increase the risk of infection and cross-contamination.

APPLICATION GUIDELINES

Dressings are applied after cleansing and debridement techniques guided by the patient assessment. Application is conducted using appropriate infection control guidelines with the clean or, at times, sterile technique. Further discussion of infection control guidelines can be found in Chapter 2. After wound bed preparation and the selection of a dressing, prepare the application area and gather the necessary supplies. Wound dressings are applied to clean, dry, intact periwound tissue. Excess body hair can affect the adherence of dressings and should be trimmed before application. Avoid shaving the area to lessen the risk of adverse reactions. The application of adherent tape sprays or liquids to the periwound tissue is not recommended but can be used with wound closure strips. Nonocclusive and occlusive dressings can remain in place over a wound for varying periods based on the type (Table 5-4). The durations are general recommendations, and clinicians should modify wear times and perform dressing changes with the development of dressing integrity issues, clinical infection, or adverse reactions. Table 5-5 provides indications for dressing changes.

Table 5-4. Dressing Wear Duration

Dressing Type	Duration in Days
Woven, nonwoven, and impregnated sterile gauze; nonadherent pads; and adhesive strips and patches	1
Wound closure strips	5-10
Alginates	≤ 7
Films and foams	3-7
Hydrogels	1-7
Hydrocolloids	5-7
Dermal adhesives	5-10

Table 5-5. Indications for Dressing Changes

- Leakage of exudate
- Excessive saturation of dressing with exudate
- Strike-through
- Separation of dressing edges from the periwound tissue
- Development of channels in dressing
- Loss of barrier capabilities/properties (occlusive dressings)
- Change in wound status during healing process
- Desiccation of wound bed
- Maceration of the wound bed and periwound tissue
- Adherence of dressing to the wound bed
- Clinical features of infection
- Clinical features of adverse reactions

Additionally, in the absence of complications, alginates, films, foams, hydrogels, and hydrocolloids can remain in place longer than the recommendations.[105] Dressing transitions may be required during the healing process based on cellular and chemical activities in the wound bed.[7-9,43,81,96,106] For example, a full-thickness abrasion can initially produce heavy amounts of exudate and require an absorbent dressing such as an alginate or foam. As healing progresses and levels of exudate decrease, the continued use of an absorbent dressing can desiccate the wound bed and delay healing. A transition to a less absorbent dressing (eg, hydrocolloid or film) is needed to maintain an optimal moist healing environment.

Nonocclusive

Woven and nonwoven sterile gauze squares and nonadherent pads used as primary dressings are removed from the sterile package and placed directly on the wound. The dressings should overlap the wound minimally on the periwound tissue to lessen the risk of maceration. These dressings will require a secondary dressing for adherence. Adhesive gauze or nonadherent, self-adherent, or

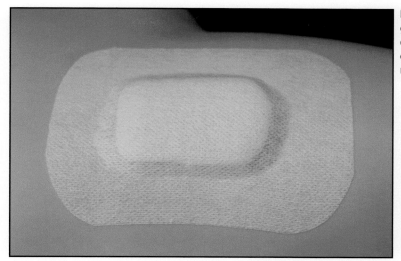

Figure 5-17. Adhesive gauze secondary dressing over a primary foam dressing on a wound model.

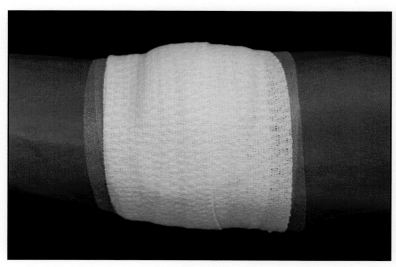

Figure 5-18. Lightweight elastic tape over pre-wrap and primary dressing.

adherent tapes and wraps can be used as secondary dressings. With intact periwound tissue and no known allergies, adhesive gauze or adherent tapes can secure the dressings. If the body area allows, extend the adhesive gauze 1 to 2 cm beyond the dressing to adhere to the periwound tissue (Figure 5-17). When using adherent tapes, cover the dressing completely. Pre-wrap can be used over the dressing before tape application (Figure 5-18). Monitor the periwound tissue for irritation with the repeated use of adhesive products. Hypoallergenic skin tapes are an alternative. Nonadherent and self-adherent wraps are bulkier but can effectively secure the primary dressing. Cover the entire dressing and slightly beyond with the wrap. Woven and nonwoven gauze squares and nonadherent pads used as secondary dressings are placed directly over the primary dressing. Clinicians can use multiple squares to absorb heavy amounts of exudate and provide protection for the wound. Adhesive gauze or nonadherent, self-adherent, or adherent tapes and wraps will be needed to secure these secondary dressings.

Woven, nonwoven, and impregnated sterile gauze strips used as primary dressings for puncture wounds are applied with sterile instruments and supplies. Table 5-6 details the guidelines for the application of the strips.

Table 5-6. Application of Woven, Nonwoven, and Impregnated Sterile Gauze Strips on a Wound Model

- Gather sterile scissors, tweezers, and/or forceps and gauze strips.
- Open the container and remove the end of the strip with tweezers or forceps (Figure 5-19).

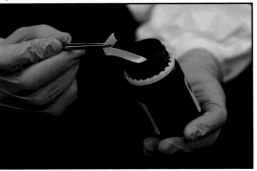

Figure 5-19

- Gently push the strip into the cavity with tweezers or forceps to loosely fill the dead space (Figure 5-20).

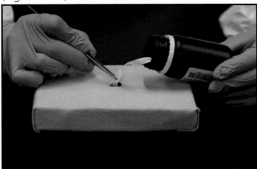

Figure 5-20

- Do not fill the cavity too tightly.
- Leave approximately 2.5 cm of the strip extending from the wound and then cut (Figure 5-21). This tail allows for removal of the strip during dressing changes.

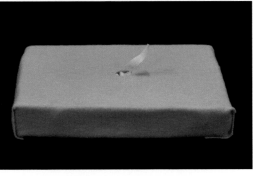

Figure 5-21

- Cover the wound bed with multiple, sterile woven or nonwoven gauze squares.
- Apply nonadherent or self-adherent wrap or hypoallergenic skin tape to cover and secure the gauze.

Adhesive strips and patches are applied as primary dressings by removing them from the packing. Place the contact layer of the dressing over the wound bed. Remove the backing from hydrocolloids and then place the dressing over the wound and periwound tissue. The dressing should overlap the wound minimally to reduce the risk of maceration. Adhesive gauze or nonadherent, self-adherent, or adherent tapes and wraps can be used as secondary dressings. Adhesive strips and patches can be used as secondary dressings applied over primary dressings to provide additional absorption, protection, and adherence.

Wound closure strips are primary dressings for tissue approximation with lacerations and incisions. See Table 5-7 for the application of wound closure strips.

Occlusive

Alginates, films, foams, hydrogels, hydrocolloids, and dermal adhesives are available in individual sterile packaging. Alginate, film, foam, hydrogel, and hydrocolloid sheet dressings are removed from the packaging and cut with clean or sterile scissors based on the wound size, shape, and location. Generally, cut these dressings 1 to 2 cm larger than the wound to extend onto the periwound tissue to provide adherence and an adequate edge seal.[6,9,67,68] Film dressings can be difficult to cut and shape to the wound. However, choose an appropriate size to extend beyond the wound bed by 1 to 2 cm. Hydrogels should be cut to the size of the wound and not extend beyond to lessen the risk of periwound maceration. Following any necessary trimming, alginates and nonadhesive foams used as primary dressings are placed directly on the wound bed and periwound tissue. Remove the backing from hydrocolloids and then place it over the wound and periwound tissue. Hydrogels as primary dressings are placed directly over the wound. Film dressings have a paper/plastic backing, and removal and application as a primary dressing must follow the manufacturer's instructions. Remove the backing pieces(s) and place the film on the wound bed and periwound tissue without tension.[9] There are several foams and hydrogels incorporated into a film secondary dressing. These dressings are applied in a similar sequence as a primary film dressing. Alginates, films, foams, hydrogels, and hydrocolloids should be applied without bunching or wrinkling, which can result in the formation of channels and subsequent leakage of exudate, compromising barrier properties (Figure 5-26). Nonadhesive alginates, foams, and hydrogels will require a secondary dressing. Films and hydrocolloids can be used as secondary dressings; films are perhaps more effective in securing the dressing and providing occlusion.[67] Several dressings are made with a small label that allows the clinician to record the date of dressing application (Figure 5-27). This dressing documentation can be helpful when multiple clinicians are involved in the management of the patient.

Dermal adhesives are primary dressings used for tissue approximation with lacerations and incisions. Clinicians should refer to applicable state practice acts before their use. See Table 5-8 for instructions on the application of dermal adhesives.

Table 5-7. Application of Wound Closure Strips on a Wound Model

- Apply a thin coat of tincture of benzoin on the periwound tissue to increase adherence of the strips, if necessary.
- Open the package and remove the card.
- Apply the strips individually (as described) or together from the card.
- Remove a strip from the card and anchor one half to the periwound tissue below the wound (Figure 5-22).

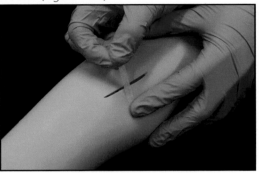

Figure 5-22

- Generally, the first strip is placed at the middle of the wound.
- Approximate the wound edges using fingers and pull the strip, without tension, across the wound (Figure 5-23).

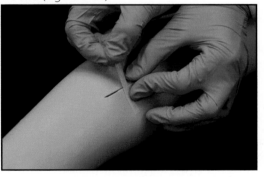

Figure 5-23

- Anchor the other half of the strip to the periwound tissue above the wound (Figure 5-24).

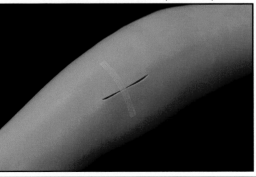

Figure 5-24

continued

Table 5-7. Application of Wound Closure Strips on a Wound Model (continued)

- Apply additional strips across the wound, approximately 3 mm apart, until approximation of the wound edges is complete (Figure 5-25).

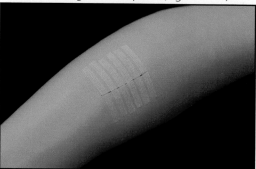

Figure 5-25

- If tissues do not approximate, carefully remove the strip over the area. Peel each side of the strip toward the wound. Reapply another strip.
- Cover the wound and strips with woven or nonwoven sterile gauze squares or nonadherent pads.
- Apply nonadherent or self-adherent wrap or hypoallergenic skin tape to cover and secure the gauze or pad.

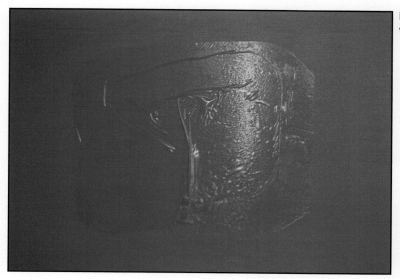

Figure 5-26. Bunching and wrinkling of a film dressing.

Figure 5-27. Label on a film dressing.

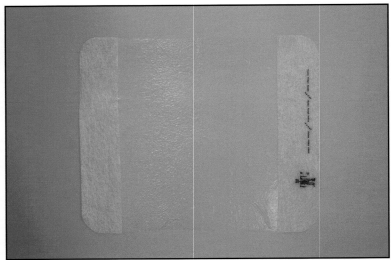

Table 5-8. Application of Dermal Adhesives on a Wound Model[84,85]

- Position the patient and wound in a horizontal position.
- Gently crush the ampoule in the middle or remove the applicator tip.
- Hold the ampoule or applicator downward and gently squeeze, allowing the adhesive to push into the tip (Figure 5-28).

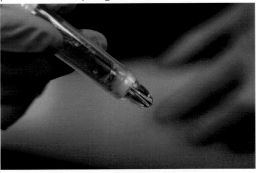

Figure 5-28

- Approximate the wound edges with fingers and slowly apply a thin layer of adhesive on the wound edges using a gentle brushing motion in a continuous layer (Figure 5-29).

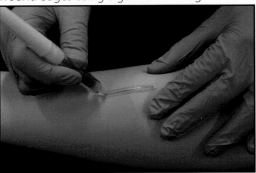

Figure 5-29

continued

Table 5-8. Application of Dermal Adhesives on a Wound Model[84,85] (continued)

- Maintain tissue approximation throughout the application process and for 60 seconds after application, allowing the adhesive to polymerize.
- Application of a second layer of adhesive is not recommended.
- Maximal adhesion should be achieved within minutes and complete polymerization when the adhesive is no longer tacky (Figure 5-30).

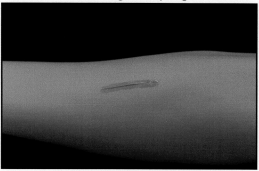

Figure 5-30

- A secondary dressing of woven or nonwoven sterile gauze squares or nonadherent pads can be applied over the wound.
- Apply nonadherent or self-adherent wrap or hypoallergenic skin tape to cover the gauze or pads.

APPLICATION PEARLS

This information focuses on suggestions for the application of wound dressings. Use these points to enhance dressing effectiveness and improve patient compliance to promote an optimal healing environment.

Consider applying an additional secondary dressing for athletes and active patients to maintain adherence of the primary dressing to the periwound tissue during practices, competitions, and recreational activities. Apply adhesive gauze to the edges of nonadhesive alginates, foams, and hydrogels adhered with a film secondary dressing, foams and hydrogels incorporated in a film secondary dressing, and film primary dressings.[40,44] Cut strips of adhesive gauze in 1 to 1.5 cm widths and lengths of the dressing (Figure 5-31). Apply half of the strip on the dressing edge and the remainder on the periwound tissue (Figure 5-32). Continue to apply a strip on each dressing edge and periwound tissue (Figure 5-33). A secondary dressing of adhesive gauze can be applied over a primary hydrocolloid dressing, extending 1 to 2 cm beyond the dressing edges (Figure 5-34). Rounding the corners of the adhesive gauze will prevent the edges from rolling on contact with clothing or equipment. If the edges of the adhesive gauze separate from the periwound tissue, trim the gauze or apply a new strip(s) or layer to maintain adherence of the dressing. Do not disturb the primary or secondary dressing during trimming. Clinicians can use nonadherent, self-adherent, or adherent tapes and wraps to cover primary and secondary dressings for additional protection. After the conclusion of the activity, remove the tapes and wraps without disturbing the dressings. Clinicians can encourage athletes to shower in-house with the tapes and wraps left in place. After showering, the clinician can remove the tapes and wraps and inspect the dressing(s). Patients can safely bathe and shower with films and hydrocolloids and alginates, foams, and hydrogels adhered with a film secondary dressing. Patients should not soak the dressings. Dressings can be lightly patted and allowed to air dry after wetting.

Figure 5-31. An adhesive gauze roll and cut strips.

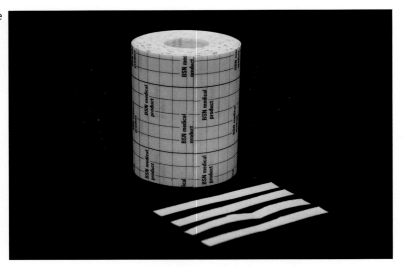

Figure 5-32. An adhesive gauze strip on a film dressing and periwound tissue.

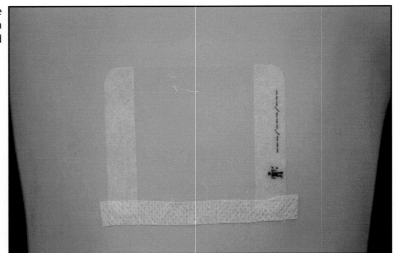

Figure 5-33. Adhesive gauze strips on the edges of a film dressing and periwound tissue.

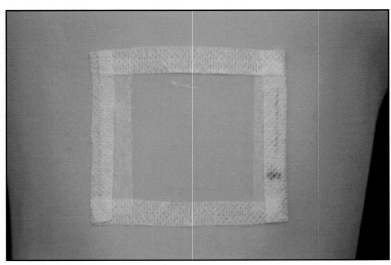

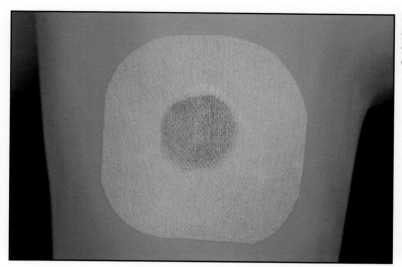

Figure 5-34. Adhesive gauze secondary dressing over a primary hydrocolloid dressing.

Several suggestions focus on the initial application and wear of occlusive dressings for athletes and active patients. Clinicians must apply occlusive dressings to dry skin to ensure edge seal and adherence to the periwound tissue. Avoid the application of occlusive dressings during practices, competitions, and activities or immediately upon conclusion. Allow the athlete or patient to shower, cool down, and cease perspiring before application. After the dressing application, a period (eg, overnight) of nonactivity will allow sufficient adherence of the dressing to the periwound tissue to withstand practices, competitions, or activity the following day. Nonocclusive dressings can be applied during activity with follow-up management in the athletic training facility. Occlusive dressings trap moisture over the wound bed. Perspiration from the activity will be trapped and cause the dressing to swell. This excess moisture should evaporate over time based on the dressing MVTR. Clinicians should monitor dressing integrity daily because moisture accumulation and swelling can saturate the dressing, increase the risk of maceration, create channels, and lead to rupture or leakage.

Several factors influence the application of dressings for finger and toe wounds. Clinicians must consider the limited periwound tissue available for dressing adherence and the functional requirements of the fingers and toes in the dressing selection, size, and application. Clinicians should manage finger and toe wounds individually with primary and secondary dressings. The dressings should cause minimal restrictions in finger and toe range of motion and tactical sensation for work and athletic activities. Clinicians can use thin-profile primary dressings such as woven and nonwoven gauze, nonadherent pads, adhesive strips and patches, films, and hydrocolloids with a secondary dressing. Select and cut (if necessary) the primary dressing. Cut a piece of adhesive gauze or lightweight elastic tape to extend from the fingertip or tip of the toe, over the dressing, and onto the periwound tissue proximally. Apply the primary dressing and then place the gauze or tape over the fingertip or tip of the toe (Figure 5-35). Adhere the sides of the gauze or tape together and to the skin, avoiding wrinkles (Figure 5-36). Trim the excess gauze or tape, leaving enough to maintain adherence on the sides (Figure 5-37). The gauze or tape can be trimmed or replaced as needed.

Some wounds and surrounding soft tissues and structures may require additional protection in combination with primary and secondary dressings. Various pads and protective devices can be applied over the dressing(s) to lessen shear and tensile forces and tensile loads. Felt or foam donut pads and nonsterile hydrogels applied over the primary or secondary dressing can reduce friction in the management of open and closed blisters (Figure 5-38). The pads or hydrogels can be anchored with adhesive gauze or nonadherent, self-adherent, or adherent tapes and wraps and carefully removed after activity, leaving the dressing(s) intact. Clinicians can also use off-the-shelf or custom-made rigid pads to protect the wound and surrounding tissues and structures.

Figure 5-35. Application of adhesive gauze over the fingertip.

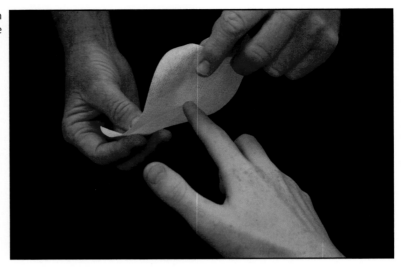

Figure 5-36. Adhesive gauze adhered to the finger.

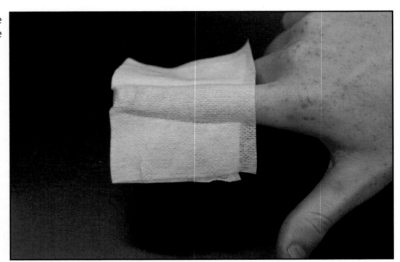

Figure 5-37. Adhesive gauze trimmed.

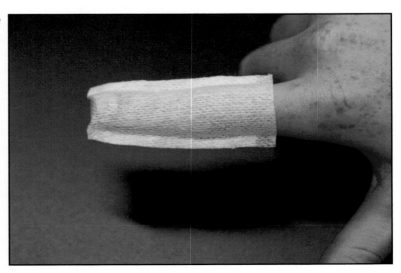

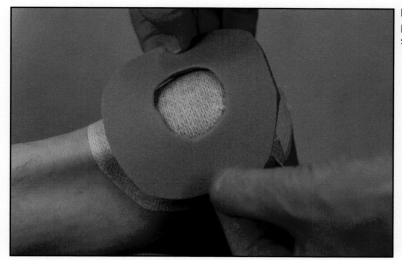

Figure 5-38. A foam donut pad over primary and secondary dressings.

SUMMARY

Nonocclusive and occlusive wound dressings are critical in the management of acute skin trauma. Dressings should create a moist healing environment, promote healing, lessen the risk of cross-contamination and infection, lessen pain, and protect the wound from further trauma. Dressings are categorized by material construction, purpose, structure, and composition and are used as primary or secondary dressings. Nonocclusive dressings include woven, nonwoven, and impregnated sterile gauze; nonadherent pads; adhesive strips and patches; and wound closure strips. Occlusive dressings consist of alginates, films, foams, hydrogels, hydrocolloids, and dermal adhesives. Characteristics of the wound, the availability of dressing materials, and patient needs and activity level will guide the selection of an appropriate dressing. Wound healing is a dynamic and changing process requiring the clinician to monitor the patient and select dressings corresponding to the wound environment, patient status, and dressing goal. Application guidelines differ based on the dressing type. Clinicians should ensure dressing integrity and adherence to enhance dressing effectiveness, increase patient compliance, and promote an environment conducive to healing.

REFERENCES

1. Ovington LG. Hanging wet-to-dry dressings out to dry. *Home Healthc Nurse.* 2001;19(8):477-483.
2. Ovington LG. The well dressed wound: An overview of dressing types. *Wounds.* 2000;10(suppl A):1A-11A.
3. Ovington LG. Dressings and skin substitutes. In: McCulloch JM, Kloth LC, eds. *Wound Healing: Evidence-Based Management.* 4th ed. F.A. Davis; 2010:180-195.
4. Winter GD. Formation of the scab and the rate of epithelialization of superficial wounds in the skin of the young domestic pig. *Nature.* 1962;193:293-294.
5. Hinman CD, Maibach H, Winter GD. Effect of air exposure and occlusion on experimental human skin wounds. *Nature.* 1963;200:377-378.
6. Kannon GA, Garrett AB. Moist wound healing with occlusive dressings: A clinical review. *Dermatol Surg.* 1995;21(7):583-590.
7. Myer A. Dressings. In: Kloth LC, McCulloch JM, eds. *Wound Healing Alternatives in Management.* 3rd ed. F.A. Davis; 2002:232-270.

8. Bolton L. Operational definition of moist wound healing. *J Wound Ostomy Continence Nurs.* 2007;34(1):23-29.

9. Myers BA. *Wound Management: Principles and Practice.* 2nd ed. Pearson Prentice Hall; 2008:123-159.

10. Bolton LL, Monte K, Pirone LA. Moisture and healing: Beyond the jargon. *Ostomy Wound Manage.* 2000;46(1A suppl):51S-62S.

11. Panuncialman J, Falanga V. The science of wound bed preparation. *Clin Plast Surg.* 2007;34(4):621-632.

12. Trudigan J. Investigating the use of aquafoam hydrogel in wound management. *Br J Nurs.* 2000;9(14):943-947.

13. Alvarez O. Moist environment for healing: Matching the dressing to the wound. *Ostomy Wound Manage.* 1988;21:64-83.

14. Baxter CR. Immunologic reactions in chronic wounds. *Am J Surg.* 1994;167(1A):12S-14S.

15. Kerstein MD. Moist wound healing: The clinical perspective. *Ostomy Wound Manage.* 1995;41(7A suppl):37S-44S.

16. Lydon MJ, Hutchinson JJ, Rippon M, et al. Dissolution of wound coagulum and promotion of granulation tissue under DuoDERM. *Wounds.* 1989;1(2):95-106.

17. Varghese MC, Balin AK, Carter M, Caldwell D. Local environment of chronic wounds under synthetic dressings. *Arch Dermatol.* 1986;122(1):52-57.

18. Witkowski JA, Parish LC. Cutaneous ulcer therapy. *Int J Dermatol.* 1986;25(7):420-426.

19. Buchan IA, Andrews JK, Lang SM, Borman JG, Harvey Kemble JV, Lamberty BGH. Clinical and laboratory investigation of the composition and properties of human skin wound exudate under semipermeable dressings. *Burns.* 1981;7(5):326-334.

20. Buchan IA, Andrews JK, Lang SM. Laboratory investigation of the composition and properties of pig skin wound exudate under Op-site. *Burns.* 1981;8(1):39-46.

21. Saymen DG, Nathan P, Holder IA, Hill EO, Macmillan BG. Control of surface wound infection: Skin versus synthetic grafts. *Appl Microbiol.* 1973;25(6):921-934.

22. Madden MR, Nolan E, Finkelstein JL, et al. Comparison of an occlusive and a semi-occlusive dressing and the effect of the wound exudate upon keratinocyte proliferation. *J Trauma.* 1989;29(7):924-930.

23. Katz MH, Alvarez AF, Kirsner RS, Eaglstein WH, Falanga V. Human wound fluid from acute wounds stimulates fibroblast and endothelial cell growth. *J Am Acad Dermatol.* 1991;25(6 Pt 1):1054-1058.

24. Eaglestein WH. Occlusive dressings. *J Dermatol Surg Oncol.* 1993;19(8):716-720.

25. Chen WY, Rogers AA, Lydon MJ. Characterization of biologic properties of wound fluid collected during early stages of wound healing. *J Invest Dermatol.* 1992;99(5):559-564.

26. Matsuoka J, Grotendorst GR. Two peptides related to platelet-derived growth factor are present in human wound fluid. *Proc Natl Acad Sci U S A.* 1989;86(12):4416-4420.

27. Alper JC, Tibbetts LL, Sarazen AAJ. The in vitro response of fibroblasts to the fluid that accumulates under a vapor-permeable membrane. *J Invest Dermatol.* 1985;84(6):513-515.

28. Eaglstein WH, Mertz PM. New methods for assessing epidermal wound healing: The effects of triamcinolone acetonide and polyethylene film occlusion. *J Invest Dermatol.* 1978;71(6):382-384.

29. Alvarez OM, Mertz PM, Eaglstein WH. The effect of occlusive dressings on collagen synthesis and re-epithelialization in superficial wounds. *J Surg Res.* 1983;35(2):142-148.

30. Bolton LL, Johnson CL, van Rijswijk L. Occlusive dressings: Therapeutic agents and effects on drug delivery. *Clin Dermatol.* 1991;9(4):573-583.

31. Jones J. Winter's concept of moist wound healing: A review of the evidence and impact on clinical practice. *J Wound Care.* 2005;14(6):273-276.

32. Jonkman MF, Hoeksma EA, Nieuwenhuis P. Accelerated epithelization under a highly vapor-permeable wound dressing is associated with increased precipitation of fibrin(ogen) and fibronectin. *J Invest Dermatol.* 1990;94(4):477-484.

33. Knighton DR, Silver IA, Hunt TK. Regulation of wound-healing angiogenesis—Effect of oxygen gradients and inspired oxygen concentration. *Surgery.* 1981;90(2):262-270.

34. Dyson M, Young S, Pendle CL, Webster DF, Lang SM. Comparison of the effects of moist and dry conditions on dermal repair. *J Invest Dermatol.* 1988;91(5):434-439.

35. Champsaur A, Amamou R, Nefzi A, Marichy J. Use of Duoderm in the treatment of skin graft donor sites. Comparative study of Duoderm and tulle gras. *Ann Chir Plast Esthet.* 1986;31(3):273-278.

36. Hermans MH, Hermans RP. Duoderm, an alternative dressing for smaller burns. *Burns Incl Therm Inj.* 1986;12(3):214-219.

37. Thomas DW, Hill CM, Lewis MA, Stephens P, Walker R, Von Der Weth A. Randomized clinical trial of the effect of semi-occlusive dressings on the microflora and clinical outcome of acute facial wounds. *Wound Repair Regen.* 2000;8(4):258-263.

38. Hultén L. Dressings for surgical wounds. *Am J Surg.* 1994;167(1A):42S-44S.

39. Rubio PA. Use of semiocclusive, transparent film dressings for surgical wound protection: Experience in 3637 cases. *Int Surg.* 1991;76(4):253-254.

40. Beam JW. Occlusive dressings and the healing of standardized abrasions. *J Athl Train.* 2008;43(6):600-607.

41. Mertz PM, Marshall DA, Eaglstein WH. Occlusive wound dressings to prevent bacterial invasion and wound infection. *J Am Acad Dermatol.* 1985;12(4):662-668.

42. Claus EE, Fusco CF, Ingram T, Ingersoll CD, Edwards JE, Melham TJ. Comparison of the effects of selected dressings on the healing of standardized abrasions. *J Athl Train.* 1998;33(2):145-149.

43. Thomas S. *A structured approach to the selection of dressings.* World Wide Wounds. 1997. Accessed November 24, 2022. http://www.worldwidewounds.com/1997/july/Thomas-Guide/Dress-Select.html

44. Beam JW. Effects of occlusive dressings on healing of partial-thickness abrasions. *Athl Train Sports Health Care.* 2012;4(2):58-66.

45. Turner T. Which dressing and why? *Nurs Times.* 1982;78(29):1-3.

46. Eriksson E, Perez N, Slama J, Page CP, Andree C, Maguire JH. Treatment of chronic, nonhealing abdominal wound in a liquid environment. *Ann Plast Surg.* 1996;36(1):80-83.

47. Vogt PM, Andree C, Breuing K, et al. Dry, moist, and wet skin wound repair. *Ann Plast Surg.* 1995;34(5):493-499.

48. Casey G. Wound dressings. *Paediatr Nurs.* 2001;13(4):39-42.

49. Lloyd L, Kennedy J, Methacanon P, Paterson M, Knill C. Carbohydrate polymers as wound management aids. *Carbohyd Polym.* 1998;37:315-322.

50. Barnett A, Berkowitz RL, Mills R, Vistnes LM. Comparison of synthetic adhesive moisture vapor permeable and fine mesh gauze dressings for split-thickness skin graft donor sites. *Am J Surg.* 1983;145(3):379-381.

51. Nelson DB, Dilloway MA. Principles, products, and practical aspects of wound care. *Crit Care Nurs Q.* 2002;25(1):33-54.

52. Jones AM, San Miguel L. Are modern wound dressings a clinical and cost-effective alternative to the use of gauze? *J Wound Care.* 2006;15(2):65-69.

53. Beam JW, Buckley B, Holcomb WR, Ciocca M. National Athletic Trainers' Association position statement: Management of acute skin trauma. *J Athl Train.* 2016;51(12):1053-1070.

54. Bradley M, Cullum N, Sheldon T. The debridement of chronic wounds: A systematic review. *Health Technol Assess.* 1999;3(17 Pt 1):1-78.

55. Singhal A, Reis ED, Kerstein MD. Options for nonsurgical debridement of necrotic wounds. *Adv Skin Wound Care.* 2001;14(2):96-100.

56. Harvey C. Wound healing. *Orthop Nurs.* 2005;24(2):143-157.

57. Cho M, Hunt TK. The overall clinical approach to wounds. In: Falanga V, ed. *Cutaneous Wound Healing.* Martin Dunitz, Ltd; 2001:141-154.

58. Bethell E. Why gauze dressings should not be the first choice to manage most acute surgical cavity wounds. *J Wound Care.* 2003;12(6):237-239.

59. Honsik KA, Romeo MW, Hawley CJ, Romeo SJ, Romeo JP. Sideline skin and wound care for acute injuries. *Curr Sports Med Rep.* 2007;6(3):147-154.

60. Farion KJ, Russell KF, Osmond MH, et al. Tissue adhesives for traumatic lacerations in children and adults. *Cochrane Database Syst Rev.* 2002;3:CD003326.

61. Dumville JC, Coulthard P, Worthington HV, et al. Tissue adhesives for closure of surgical incisions. *Cochrane Database Syst Rev.* 2014;11:CD004287.

62. Cannon BC, Cannon JP. Management of pressure ulcers. *Am J Health Syst Pharm.* 2004;61(18):1895-1905.

63. Piacquadio D, Nelson DB. Alginates. A "new" dressing alternative. *J Dermatol Surg Oncol.* 1992;18(11):992-995.

64. Hess CT, Kirsner RS. Orchestrating wound healing: Assessing and preparing the wound bed. *Adv Skin Wound Care.* 2003;16(5):246-257.

65. Wiechula R. The use of moist wound-healing dressings in the management of split-thickness skin graft donor sites: A systematic review. *Int J Nurs Pract.* 2003;9(2):S9-S17.

66. Chaby G, Senet P, Vaneau M, et al. Dressings for acute and chronic wounds: A systematic review. *Arch Dermatol.* 2007;143(10):1297-1304.

67. Fonder MA, Mamelak AJ, Lazarus GS, Chanmugam A. Occlusive wound dressings in emergency medicine and acute care. *Emerg Med Clin North Am.* 2007;25(1):235-242.

68. Hom DB, Adams G, Koreis M, Maisel R. Choosing the optimal dressing for irradiated soft tissue wounds. *Otolaryngol Head Neck Surg.* 1999;121(5):591-598.

69. Dumville JC, Gray TA, Walter CJ, et al. Dressings for the prevention of surgical site infection. *Cochrane Database Syst Rev.* 2016;12:CD003091.

70. Ma KK, Chan MF, Pang SM. The effectiveness of using a lipido-colloid dressing for patients with traumatic digital wounds. *Clin Nurs Res.* 2006;15(2):119-134.

71. Falanga V. Occlusive wound dressings. Why, when, which? *Arch Dermatol.* 1988;124(6):872-877.

72. Hollander JE, Singer AJ. Laceration management. *Ann Emerg Med.* 1999;34(3):356-367.

73. Wijetunge DB. Management of acute and traumatic wounds: Main aspects of care in adults and children. *Am J Surg.* 1994;167(1A):56S-60S.

74. Ameen H, Moore K, Lawrence JC, Harding KG. Investigating the bacterial barrier properties of four contemporary wound dressings. *J Wound Care.* 2000;9(8):385-388.

75. Bowler PG, Delargy H, Prince D, Fondberg L. The viral barrier properties of some occlusive dressings and their role in infection control. *Wounds.* 1993;5(1):1-8.

76. Atiyeh BS, Ioannovich J, Al Amm CA, El Musa KA. Management of acute and chronic open wounds: The importance of moist environment in optimal wound healing. *Curr Pharm Biotechnol.* 2002;3(3):179-195.

77. Cohen KI, Diegelmann R, Yager D, Wornum II, Graham M, Crossland M. Wound care and wound healing. In: Spencer S, Galloway D, eds. *Principles of Surgery.* International ed. McGraw-Hill Book Company; 1999:269-290.

78. Vermeulen H, van Hattem JM, Storm-Versloot MN, Ubbink DT, Westerbos SJ. Topical silver for treating infected wounds. *Cochrane Database Syst Rev.* 2007;1:CD005486.

79. Choucair M, Phillips T. A review of wound healing and dressings material. *Skin Ageing.* 1998;6:37-43.

80. Thomas S, Hay P. Fluid handling properties of hydrogel dressings. *Ostomy Wound Manage.* 1995;41(3):54-56, 58-59.

81. Eisenbud D, Hunter H, Kessler L, Zulkowski K. Hydrogel wound dressings: Where do we stand in 2003? *Ostomy Wound Manage.* 2003;49(10):52-57.

82. Thomas S, Loveless P. *A comparative study of the properties of twelve hydrocolloid dressings.* World Wide Wounds. July 1997. Accessed November 24, 2022. http://www.worldwidewounds.com/1997/july/Thomas-Hydronet/hydronet.html

83. Hess CT. When to use hydrocolloid dressings. *Adv Skin Wound Care.* 2000;13(2):63-64.

84. Dermabond Advanced instructions for use. Ethicon. Accessed November 23, 2022. https://www.jnjmedicaldevices.com/en-US/product/dermabond-advanced-topical-skin-adhesive

85. Histoacryl Clear & Blue topical skin adhesive. TissueSeal. Accessed November 23, 2022. http://tissueseal.com/wp-content/uploads/2020/02/Histoacryl_Clear_Blue_IFU.pdf

86. Perron AD, Garcia JA, Hays EP, Schafermeyer R. The efficacy of cyanoacrylate-derived surgical adhesive for use in the repair of lacerations during competitive athletics. *Am J Emerg Med.* 2000;18(3):261-263.

87. Branfield AS. Use of tissue adhesives in sport? A new application in international ice hockey. *Br J Sports Med.* 2004;38(1):95-96.

88. Davidson JM. Animal models for wound repair. *Arch Dermatol Res.* 1998;290(suppl):S1-S11.

89. Storm-Versloot MN, Vos CG, Ubbink DT, Vermeulen H. Topical silver for preventing wound infection. *Cochrane Database Syst Rev.* 2010;3:CD006478.

90. Bergin S, Wraight P. Silver based wound dressings and topical agents for treating diabetic foot ulcers. *Cochrane Database Syst Rev.* 2006;1:CD005082.

91. Heffernan A, Martin AJ. A comparison of a modified form of Granuflex (Granuflex Extra Thin) and a conventional dressing in the management of lacerations, abrasions and minor operation wounds in an accident and emergency department. *J Accid Emerg Med.* 1994;11(4):227-230.

92. Hutchinson JJ, McGuckin M. Occlusive dressings: A microbiologic and clinical review. *Am J Infect Control.* 1990;18(4):257-268.

93. Hermans MH. Clinical benefit of a hydrocolloid dressing in closed surgical wounds. *J ET Nurs.* 1993;20(2):68-72.

94. Motta GJ. Dressed for success: How moisture-retentive dressings promote healing. *Nursing.* 1993;23(12):26-33.

95. Barr J. Physiology of healing: The basis for the principles of wound management. *Medsurg Nurs.* 1995;4(5):387-392.

96. Ayello EA, Dowsett C, Schultz GS, et al. TIME heals all wounds. *Nursing.* 2004;34(4):36-41.

97. Lawrence JC, Lilly HA. Are hydrocolloid dressings bacteria proof? *Pharm J.* 1987;239:184.

98. Kearney MT, Duncan ER, Kahn M, Wheatcroft SB. Insulin resistance and endothelial cell dysfunction: Studies in mammalian models. *Exp Physiol.* 2008;93(1):158-163.

99. Patterson GK, Martindale RG. Nutrition and wound healing. In: McCulloch JM, Kloth LC, eds. *Wound Healing: Evidence-Based Management.* 4th ed. F.A. Davis; 2010:44-50.

100. Ehrlich HP, Hunt TK. Effects of cortisone and vitamin A on wound healing. *Ann Surg.* 1968;167(3):324-328.

101. Ponec M, de Haas C, Bachra BN, Polano MK. Effects of glucocorticosteroids on primary human skin fibroblasts. I. Inhibition of the proliferation of cultured primary human skin and mouse L929 fibroblasts. *Arch Dermatol Res (1975).* 1977;259(2):117-123.

102. Salcido RS. Do anti-inflammatories have a role in wound healing? *Adv Skin Wound Care.* 2005;18(2):65-66.

103. Telfer NR, Moy RL. Drug and nutrient aspects of wound healing. *Dermatol Clin.* 1993;11(4):729-737.

104. Busti AJ, Hooper JS, Amaya CJ, Kazi S. Effects of preoperative anti-inflammatory and immunomodulating therapy on surgical wound healing. *Pharmocotherapy.* 2005;25(11):1566-1591.

105. Nemeth AJ, Eaglstein WH, Taylor JR, Peerson LJ, Falanga V. Faster healing and less pain in skin biopsy sites treated with an occlusive dressing. *Arch Dermatol.* 1991;127(11):1679-1683.

106. Ennis WJ, Meneses P. Complications in repair. In: McCulloch JM, Kloth LC, eds. *Wound Healing: Evidence-Based Management.* 4th ed. F.A. Davis; 2010:51-64.

6

MONITORING AND EDUCATION

Following cleansing, debridement, and dressing interventions, the management of acute skin trauma requires the clinician to monitor and educate the patient. Reassessment of the patient and wound evaluates the effectiveness of the interventions, identifies the development of adverse reactions, and guides the management plan. Patient education and adherence to the management plan are necessary to promote healing and optimal function. This chapter discusses daily monitoring and reassessment of the patient and wound, the importance of patient education during healing, and patient adherence to the management plan. The chapter begins with the monitoring process to reassess the patient, wound bed, periwound tissue, and dressing. The role and components of patient education are presented next. The chapter concludes with strategies to enhance patient adherence to the management plan.

DOI: 10.1201/9781003523055-6

Table 6-1. Reassessment Findings Requiring Referral[1-3]
• Lack of progress in the expected rate of healing
• Negative lifestyle behaviors
• Inadequate diet and nutrition
• Noncompliance with medications
• Comorbidities
• Nonadherence to the management plan
• Clinical features of infection
• Clinical features of adverse reactions

MONITORING AND REASSESSMENT

Monitoring and reassessment of the patient and wound are paramount in the management of acute skin trauma. Clinicians should monitor patients daily. The athletic setting typically allows for daily contact with most athletes in the athletic training facility. In cases that do not allow daily monitoring, clinicians should reassess the patient regularly. Monitoring and reassessment verify the effects of cleansing, debridement, and dressing interventions on wound healing and patient functional goals; identify the clinical features associated with the development of infection and adverse reactions; and guide dressing changes and modifications to the management plan.

Monitoring is guided by the initial assessment and includes a reassessment of the patient, wound bed, periwound tissue, and dressing. The reassessment consists of those parameters from the secondary survey described in Chapter 1. The clinician will determine the extent, complexity, and parameters to reassess based on individual patient history, status, and response to the interventions and management plan. Patients who returned to athletic or work activities without restrictions immediately after injury, are asymptomatic, and present with full functional ability at the reassessment may not require a comprehensive range of motion evaluation, functional testing, neurologic and vascular screening, and review of systems. In this situation, the clinician can obtain information from the patient through open-ended questions or observation. Based on the interventions and management plan, some factors can be difficult to evaluate during the reassessment. For example, if signs and symptoms of adverse reactions and dressing integrity issues are not demonstrated, a foam dressing applied 2 days prior may remain over the wound, preventing inspection of the wound bed. Clinicians should avoid unnecessary dressing changes during reassessments and follow recommended dressing wear durations. If changes are necessary at the reassessment, monitor dressing adherence to the wound bed. Moisten the dressing with normal saline or tap water irrigation before removal to lessen the risk of further damage. Acute skin trauma progresses through an orderly reparative process. Reassessments that reveal findings inconsistent with expected outcomes are indications for re-evaluation of the management plan and consideration of patient referral. See Table 6-1 for reassessment findings that require referrals.

Patient

Patient reassessment encompasses questioning and evaluation of the patient in a holistic manner. The reassessment includes the evaluation of changes in medical history and history and the status of the present injury since the initial assessment. For example, is the patient currently taking a medication that may adversely affect healing or developing an allergy that may result in sensitivity to materials in a dressing? Changes in the location and type of pain or the development of fever may indicate the progression of infection. The reassessment of range of motion and functional status can determine the effectiveness of the interventions. For example, a patient with a full-thickness lateral proximal forearm abrasion should demonstrate a reduction in pain and an improvement in the elbow or wrist range of motion after the creation of a moist wound environment. A moist wound and dressing surface produced with occlusion prevents desiccation of nerve endings, lessens signal transduction from exposed nerve fibers, and prevents further trauma to decrease pain.[4-7] Clinicians may consider dressing modifications with patients who initially returned to activity or work and now demonstrate reductions in functional ability on reassessment. For example, a cabinet carpenter with a partial-thickness dorsal hand laceration with a hydrocolloid primary dressing and nonadherent wrap secondary dressing cannot properly grip hand tools because of the bulk of the wrap. The clinician can replace the nonadherent wrap with lower-profile adhesive gauze to allow full finger and thumb range of motion and gripping. Clinicians should perform neurologic, vascular, and review of systems reassessments for patients with initial presentation of deep wounds involving subcutaneous tissue, bone, or tendon or nerve injury; comorbidities; a history of delayed wound healing or complications; or clinical features of infection or adverse reactions. The last reassessment parameter is patient adherence to the management plan. Further discussion of patient adherence follows in the chapter.

Wound Bed

Reassessment of the wound bed involves inspection of the wound size, exudate level, odor, tissue color, and hydration. Dressing removal is required with most dressings to evaluate the wound bed. Film and hydrogel dressings allow for partial inspection of the wound bed while in place. The wound length, width, depth, and closure method will determine the rate and time to complete healing. Because objective measurements (eg, direct measurement and photography) of acute wounds are rarely performed, a subjective evaluation should reveal reduced wound length, width, and depth as healing progresses. For example, deep wounds with tissue loss require greater time to heal than superficial-thickness wounds based on the growth of new tissue and repair of the defect.[8] Wound edges approximated and closed by primary closure with dermal adhesives, wound closure strips, sutures, or staples contract and heal faster than wounds closed by secondary closure. If a wound is not demonstrating reductions in length, width, or depth as expected or dehisced, reassessment of the management plan and possible referral are indicated. Quantifying the amount of exudate can be difficult during the reassessment. Exudate levels should decrease as healing progresses based on cellular and chemical changes in the wound bed.[9] Exudate amounts can be determined with an evaluation of the dressing. For example, dressing saturation or integrity or barrier issues (eg, strike-through, channel formation, or leakage) can result from the production of heavy exudate. Excess exudate production can be associated with the depth of tissue damage, wound size, infection, and inappropriate dressing use. Exudate color can indicate the status of the wound and the progression of healing. **Serous** drainage is produced during the inflammatory stage of healing and is clear and watery in appearance. **Sanguineous** drainage, identified with small amounts of blood, is also present in the inflammatory stage. Thin, watery, and pink **serosanguinous** drainage is normal in most wounds. **Purulent** drainage is identified as thick and milky with a tan, yellow, gray, green, or brown color and can be associated with infection. Heavy production of exudate and the presence of purulent drainage warrant referral and re-evaluation of the management plan and dressing interventions. The odor of the wound bed can be reassessed with dressing changes after cleansing of the wound bed. Wound bed odor may indicate the presence of microorganisms in the wound[10] and requires further evaluation. The color of the wound bed can determine the type and viability of the tissue, progression of healing, and effectiveness of the interventions.[11,12] Cleansing the wound bed is necessary to remove dressing residue and exudate to allow for unobstructed inspection. Most acute

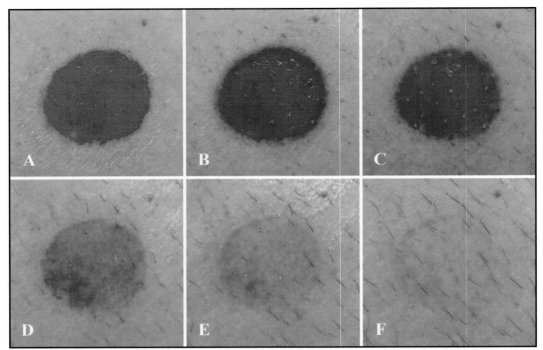

Figure 6-1. Wound bed color of a partial-thickness abrasion by day after injury. Abrasion was covered with an occlusive hydrocolloid dressing. (A) Day 1, (B) day 3, (C) day 5, (D) day 7, (E) day 10, and (F) day 14.

wounds are initially bright red, indicating viable granulation tissue. The wound color will change from bright red to pale pink as healing progresses (Figure 6-1). Tissue colors of white, yellow, tan, brown, or black indicate nonviable, devitalized slough or eschar (see Table 1-1). The presence of slough or eschar requires changes to the management plan and further evaluation. Wounds should remain hydrated throughout healing. As discussed in Chapter 5, a moist wound environment promotes healing and lessens the risk of infection. A dry wound can result in crust formation and cause delayed healing.[13] A too wet wound can also delay healing and cause maceration of the wound bed and periwound tissue.[14,15] Clinicians must be able to match the appropriate dressing to the characteristics of the wound to create and maintain a moist healing environment.

Periwound Tissue

The periwound tissue is reassessed for condition, color, and temperature. Reassessments can be conducted with the dressing over the wound or removed. Dressing removal is warranted for patients presenting with clinical features of adverse reactions. Ecchymosis, swelling, erythema, and denuded tissue in the periwound tissue are common after the initial injury. For example, tension and shear force against a hard surface can result in a laceration and contusion to the periwound tissue. During reassessments, a reduction in ecchymosis, swelling, and erythema, and healing of denuded tissue should be demonstrated. Persistent erythema or swelling can be associated with inflammation, infection, or adverse reactions such as dermatitis, requiring referral. The presence of multiple red papules at the base of hair follicles is a clinical feature of folliculitis. Folliculitis can result from occlusive dressings and in areas covered by the dressing.[1] Periwound tissue shaved before dressing application can be a contributing factor.[1] Clinicians should remove the causative dressing and refer the patient for further evaluation. Excessive exudate and the inability of dressings to manage the moisture can cause maceration of the periwound tissue. Maceration presents with soft, moist, white color skin extending from the wound bed. Clinicians can find dressing integrity and barrier issues with the production of heavy exudate. Removal of the dressing, re-evaluation of dressing choice, and possible referral are required. Clinicians can compare the temperature of the periwound tissue to the surrounding tissue. An elevated temperature can be associated with inflammation or infection. Frequent changes of adhesive primary or secondary dressings can result in trauma to the periwound tissue. Adhesives can strip or remove the epidermis, producing a wound akin to a superficial-thickness abrasion. Alternative dressing interventions may be necessary to manage epidermal damage.

Dressing

Reassessment of the dressing will identify integrity, barrier, and absorbency properties and reactions to interventions and guide dressing changes. The integrity, barrier, and absorbency properties will influence performance and healing outcomes.[1] At inspection, the primary dressing should be intact over the wound and some (eg, film or hydrocolloid) adhered to the periwound tissue. The secondary dressing should cover the primary dressing and periwound tissue if applicable. Inspect the primary dressing for wrinkling or bunching that may result from inappropriate application, tension, or friction. Dressings applied over or near a joint are subject to increased tension during athletic and work activities. Dressings over body areas covered by athletic or work uniforms or protective equipment undergo tension and friction forces during activities. Wrinkling and bunching can promote the formation of channels extending from the wound bed to the dressing edge. Increased tension and friction can also result in the separation of the dressing edges from the periwound tissue. Excessive exudate production, delayed dressing changes, or inappropriate dressing use can lead to saturation of the dressing and strike-through. The separation of dressing edges from the periwound tissue, saturation, or strike-through can result in the leakage of exudate.[13,16,17] The leakage of exudate and compromise of dressing barrier properties can increase the risk of cross-contamination, infection, and wound desiccation.[16,18,19] The clinician should consider dressing changes and reassessment of the dressing choice in the management plan. As a moist wound environment is created under film and hydrogel dressings, a brownish fluid will be visible over the wound bed. Without other clinical features, this fluid is normal and should not be confused with infection.[20] The gel produced by alginate and hydrocolloid dressings over the wound can have a foul odor. An odor in an asymptomatic patient should not be mistaken for infection.[13,21] The clinician can consider dressing changes to lessen the odor. Documentation of dressing wear duration will guide changes in the absence of integrity, barrier, and absorbency issues; adverse reactions; or infection.[1] See Table 5-4 for dressing wear durations. Clinicians should avoid unnecessary dressing changes and disturbance of the moist wound healing environment. Findings from the patient, wound bed, and periwound tissue reassessments are used in dressing transition choices during healing.

PATIENT EDUCATION AND ADHERENCE

Patient education on management plan interventions and adherence to the plan are essential to promote healing, lessen the risk of adverse events, and allow a functional return to activity. Clinicians must provide patients with clear complete instructions, explanations, and rationale for each intervention in the plan. The level of the information supplied should match the patient's current knowledge base and understanding regarding the interventions and management plan. Clinicians must ensure that the patient understands and is comfortable with the plan to achieve adherence and healing outcomes.

Education

The components of education are individualized to the patient and based on the assessment findings, patient characteristics, and management plan. Patient history obtained from the initial assessment can reveal several components clinicians should address. A history of malnutrition requires patient education on adequate dietary requirements and the importance of proper nutritional habits in the healing process. Although most patients with acute skin trauma present with diets sufficient in carbohydrate, protein, fat, water, mineral, and vitamin intake required for active lifestyles, some patients may need a referral. Patients prescribed and taking medications should receive information on the benefits, side effects, and possible implications of the medications on wound healing from a physician. Comorbid illnesses and conditions among patients require guidance and education on the impact the condition could have on healing outcomes, such as delayed healing or increased risk of infection possibly associated with diabetes.[22] Lifestyle education and referral to appropriate programs for modification consideration are needed with a history of smoking and excess alcohol use because these behaviors can impair wound healing and cause health problems. Patients with healthy, active lifestyles may also require education and temporary modifications. For example, a softball center fielder with a superficial-thickness lateral lower leg abrasion treated with a film dressing should be counseled to avoid sliding during the week of practice to prevent dislodging the dressing and allow healing to progress. For weekend games, a secondary dressing or secondary dressing and pad can be applied for additional protection during sliding movements. A triathlete with a partial-thickness plantar foot open blister caused by wearing new orthotics is treated with an occlusive dressing. The clinician can temporarily modify cardiovascular training by replacing running with an upper body ergometer or stationary cycle program to lessen shear and tensile forces and tensile loads on the wound and dressing.

Proper education on the management plan includes the goals, intervention guidelines, home care, and patient self-monitoring. With the initial assessment and management interventions, clinicians should provide education and clear explanations of plan goals to the patient. These goals, achieving rapid healing, providing optimal function, and lessening adverse events, are discussed with the patient to promote understanding and cooperation with the plan. Clinicians should educate the patient on why interventions are selected and how interventions will support the goals at levels congruent with the patient's current knowledge base. Many patients have been told and believe acute wounds should be left uncovered and allowed to breathe. The subsequent formation of eschar and exposure to the external environment are thought to be requirements for normal healing. Although acute skin trauma often heals regardless of interventions, clinicians must educate patients on the appropriate wound environment and interventions necessary to achieve the management plan goals. For most patients, a moist wound bed is an appropriate environment. Occlusive dressings and a moist wound environment are new paradigms among many patients. This idea will require explanations on why occlusive dressings are selected, how they create a moist wound environment, and the benefits of moist wound healing to promote healing, lessen the risk of infection and adverse reactions, and allow optimal function. Clinicians should emphasize the guidelines for occlusive dressing wear to prevent unnecessary dressing changes.[1] Occlusive dressings can remain over the wound bed for longer periods than nonocclusive dressings. Patients should be counseled on the length of wear, why the dressing should not be removed, and the implications of early removal. The clinician should educate the patient on changes in the wound and dressing (eg, brownish color of the wound fluid, swelling of the dressing, and odor) that may occur with the production of a moist environment. Based on the wound and complexity of the interventions, the clinician can educate the patient on how to perform home care. Clinicians should explain procedures for home care with complete instructions and rationale with real or perceived barriers addressed. Providing the patient with written instructions or demonstrating the intervention procedures can assist in the proper performance of the technique. For example, a patient with a laceration closed with sutures may need instruction on secondary dressing changes. Clinicians can use the application guidelines for woven or nonwoven sterile gauze, nonadherent pads, and self-adherent or adherent tapes and wraps found in Chapter 5 to demonstrate the technique with the patient. Clinicians must encourage patients to strictly follow the guidelines for daily self-monitoring and identifying the development of adverse events. Patients must be educated on the clinical features of infection and adverse reactions associated with interventions such as allergic contact dermatitis, folliculitis, maceration, or dressing integrity issues (eg, saturation, strike-through, or leakage). Further discussion of the causes and clinical features of infection and adverse reactions can be found in Chapter 7. Patients must understand the importance of reporting adverse events to the clinician in a timely manner and the consequences of failing to notify the clinician of signs and symptoms or dressing failure.

Adherence

A management plan with evidence-based interventions, daily monitoring and reassessment, and education can fail to achieve healing outcomes if the patient is nonadherent to the plan, guidelines, and overall goals. Clinicians begin to build and foster patient adherence during the initial assessment through communication and education. Patient adherence to the management plan can be influenced by multiple factors, such as past experiences with skin trauma and interventions, minimal education and guidelines to perform a task, or lack of clinician-patient communication.[23] Patients can present with prior wound and healing experiences that affect their actions and adherence to the current management plan.[23] For example, a patient sustained an abrasion 7 months ago and did not cover the wound with a dressing, producing increased levels of pain and delayed healing. This patient now suffers another abrasion and believes they will experience a similar level of pain and healing period despite appropriate cleansing, debridement, and dressing interventions. Clinicians should counsel the patient that prior experiences have a minimal effect on the outcomes of the current injury.[23] Clinicians can empower patients with the knowledge to recognize their control and actions with the management plan and interventions to improve adherence. Communicating and educating patients on interventions, goals, and expectations can improve adherence and lessen adverse outcomes. For example, a patient did not receive specific guidance on self-monitoring their dressing over a weekend. The primary dressing becomes saturated, and the edges separate from the periwound tissue, resulting in leakage. When the patient returns for reassessment the following week, the clinician finds the wound desiccated and the dressing adhered to the wound bed. Consider a patient given incomplete instructions regarding dressing wear duration. The patient is treated with primary film and secondary self-adherent wrap dressings and confuses the daily change of the wrap with the film dressing. The patient changes the film dressing daily, resulting in unnecessary changes that delay healing and increase the risk of infection. The clinician must also recognize barriers to task performance and create solutions to enhance adherence.[24] Clinicians can lower financial barriers by providing the patient with the supplies required to complete the intervention. For example, adhesive gauze or nonadherent, self-adherent, or adherent tapes and wraps can be provided to the patient to change secondary dressings between reassessments. Cooperation, active participation, and adherence to the management plan are vital to the patient's health and the effectiveness of the interventions on healing and functional outcomes. Providing communication with clear instructions, explanations, and rationale for interventions; demonstrating tasks and techniques; discussing patient expectations; and developing written instructions may increase patient knowledge, confidence, and adherence.[25-27]

SUMMARY

Patient monitoring and education are necessary throughout the healing process. Daily reassessments of the patient, wound bed, periwound tissue, and dressing provide the clinician with information on the effectiveness of interventions, the associated patient responses, and the development of infection and adverse events. Clinicians use these findings to assess healing and guide the management plan with changes or modifications to interventions as needed. Patient education through clear communication, instructions, and rationale is vital to promote healing, lessen adverse events, and return the patient to activity. The components of education are based on assessment findings, patient characteristics, and interventions and should include counseling on the management plan goals, intervention guidelines, home care procedures, and self-monitoring. Patient adherence to the management plan and interventions is based on effective communication and education provided by the clinician. Factors that may cause poor adherence must be recognized and addressed through education to facilitate patient understanding and cooperation.

REFERENCES

1. Beam JW, Buckley B, Holcomb WR, Ciocca M. National Athletic Trainers' Association position statement: Management of acute skin trauma. *J Athl Train*. 2016;51(12):1053-1070.
2. Myers BA. *Wound Management: Principles and Practice*. Pearson Prentice Hall; 2008:25-37.
3. Lampe KE. The general evaluation. In: McCulloch JM, Kloth LC, eds. *Wound Healing: Evidence-Based Management*. 4th ed. F.A. Davis; 2010:65-93.
4. Field CK, Kerstein MD. Overview of wound healing in a moist environment. *Am J Surg*. 1994;167(1A):2S-6S.
5. Nemeth AJ, Eaglstein WH, Taylor JR, Peerson LJ, Falanga V. Faster healing and less pain in skin biopsy sites treated with an occlusive dressing. *Arch Dermatol*. 1991;127(11):1679-1683.
6. Hermanson A, Dalsgaard CJ, Björklund H, Lindblom U. Sensory reinnervation and sensibility after superficial skin wounds in human patients. *Neurosci Lett*. 1987;74(3):377-382.
7. Dalsgaard CJ, Rydh M, Haegerstrand A. Cutaneous innervation in man visualized with protein gene product 9.5 (PGP 9.5) antibodies. *Histochemistry*. 1989;92(5):385-390.
8. Myers BA. *Wound Management: Principles and Practice*. Pearson Prentice Hall; 2008:11-24.
9. Thomas S. *A structured approach to the selection of dressings*. World Wide Wounds. 1997. Accessed March 12, 2022. http://www.worldwidewounds.com/1997/july/Thomas-Guide/Dress-Select.html
10. Hess CT, Kirsner RS. Orchestrating wound healing: Assessing and preparing the wound bed. *Adv Skin Wound Care*. 2003;16(5):246-257.
11. Bulstrode LJK, Goode AW, Scott PJ. Stereophotogrammetry for measuring rates of cutaneous healing: A comparison with conventional techniques. *Clin Sci (Lond)*. 1986;71:437-443.
12. Ferrell BA. The Sessing Scale for measurement of pressure ulcer healing. *Adv Wound Care*. 1997;10:78-80.
13. Myers BA. *Wound Management: Principles and Practice*. Pearson Prentice Hall; 2008:123-159.
14. Ovington LG. Dressings and skin substitutes. In: McCulloch JM, Kloth LC, eds. *Wound Healing: Evidence-Based Management*. 4th ed. F.A. Davis; 2010:180-195.
15. Kerstein MD. Moist wound healing: The clinical perspective. *Ostomy Wound Manage*. 1995;41(7A suppl):37S-44S.
16. Mertz PM, Marshall DA, Eaglstein WH. Occlusive wound dressings to prevent bacterial invasion and wound infection. *J Am Acad Dermatol*. 1985;12(4):662-668.

17. Myer A. Dressings. In: Kloth LC, McCulloch JM, eds. *Wound Healing Alternatives in Management*. 3rd ed. F.A. Davis; 2002:232-270.

18. Ameen H, Moore K, Lawrence JC, Harding KG. Investigating the bacterial barrier properties of four contemporary wound dressings. *J Wound Care*. 2000;9(8):385-388.

19. Bowler PG, Delargy H, Prince D, Fondberg L. The viral barrier properties of some occlusive dressings and their role in infection control. *Wounds*. 1993;5(1):1-8.

20. Alvarez O. Moist environment for healing: Matching the dressing to the wound. *Ostomy Wound Manage*. 1988;21:64-83.

21. Kannon GA, Garrett AB. Moist wound healing with occlusive dressings: A clinical review. *Dermatol Surg*. 1995;21(7):583-590.

22. Kearney MT, Duncan ER, Kahn M, Wheatcroft SB. Insulin resistance and endothelial cell dysfunction: Studies in mammalian models. *Exp Physiol*. 2008;93(1):158-163.

23. Myers BA. *Wound Management: Principles and Practice*. Pearson Prentice Hall; 2008:196-213.

24. Aljasem L, Peyrot M, Wissow L, Rubin R. The impact of barriers and self-efficacy on self-care behaviors in type 2 diabetes. *Diabetes Educ*. 2001;27:393-404.

25. Henry KD, Rosemond C, Eckert LB. Effect of number of home exercises on compliance and performance in adults over 65 years of age. *Phys Ther*. 1999;79:270-277.

26. Krichbaum K, Aarestad V, Buethe M. Exploring the connection between self-efficacy and effective diabetes self-management. *Diabetes Educ*. 2003;29:653-662.

27. Skelly AH, Arcury TA, Snively BM, et al. Self-monitoring of blood glucose in a multiethnic population of rural older adults with diabetes. *Diabetes Educ*. 2005;31:84-90.

7

INFECTIONS AND ADVERSE REACTIONS

Mario Ciocca, MD

The skin is an effective barrier preventing pathogens from entering the skin and soft tissues. Although most acute skin trauma heals uneventfully, the barrier can be disrupted, and proper wound management is needed to optimize healing and help prevent skin and soft tissue infection. Management interventions used for acute wounds can cause the development of systematic and local adverse reactions. Clinicians must monitor the patient and wound throughout healing for the clinical features of infection and adverse reactions. This chapter begins with a review of the causes and clinical features of infection. Treatment and prevention of infection are presented next. This is followed by a discussion of the etiology of adverse reactions and treatment and prevention interventions. Finally, this chapter presents criteria for patient referral to a physician in the management of acute skin trauma.

DOI: 10.1201/9781003523055-7

INFECTION

Acute skin trauma damages the skin barrier and allows microorganisms to penetrate the deeper tissue layers.[1] Infection is the most common cause of impaired wound healing.[2] The wound becomes contaminated with bacteria after disruption of the dermis, epidermis, subcutaneous tissue, or all 3. Although bacteria are present, the multiplication of organisms has yet to take place.[2] Colonization of the wound occurs when microorganisms multiply and is a normal state in tissue, producing no host reaction and no clinical features of tissue damage. Colonization of the wound may enhance rather than delay healing. Healing starts to become impaired when colonization progresses to critical colonization. Critical colonization is the transition state to invasive wound infection. During this stage, the wound is unable to maintain the balance of organisms seen at colonization, and the wound starts to appear unhealthy, but there is no tissue invasion. The reparative process of healing can pause, causing delayed healing. Infection occurs when host defenses are overwhelmed by the multiplying bacteria resulting in host injury.[2]

Types of Infection

Skin and soft tissue infections can present in a variety of ways. Purulent infections include folliculitis, furuncles, carbuncles, and abscesses. Folliculitis is a superficial infection of the hair follicles with purulence in the epidermis (Figure 7-1). An abscess refers to a collection of pus that is within the dermis and subcutaneous space (Figure 7-2). A furuncle is an extension of the hair follicle infection with a small subcutaneous abscess, and a carbuncle is a cluster of furuncles.[3,4] **Nonpurulent** infections of the skin include erysipelas, impetigo, and cellulitis. Erysipelas is a superficial infection characterized by a tender, erythematous plaque with well-demarcated borders. Impetigo is also superficial and characterized by yellow to red pustules or vesicles progressing to crusting or **bullae** (Figure 7-3).[3,4] Cellulitis is a deep dermal and subcutaneous infection. It is characterized by poorly demarcated erythema, warmth, edema, and tenderness (Figure 7-4). Cellulitis may also cause dilated and **edematous** skin lymphatics. There may be bullae formation, erythematous streaks, and tender **lymphadenopathy**.[4] A more aggressive infection that is life-threatening is necrotizing fasciitis. This infection of the subcutaneous tissue spreads along the fascial planes and is rapidly progressive and destructive. Clinical features may include edema, skin necrosis, bullae, skin discoloration, skin anesthesia, fever, or crepitus. Patients will have exacerbated pain that is out of proportion to the clinical findings.[3,4]

Causes of Infection

Streptococci bacteria are the most likely cause of nonpurulent skin and soft tissue infections. Purulent skin and soft tissue infections are more commonly caused by *Staphylococcus aureus*.[3] Cellulitis is one of the most common skin and soft tissue infections. The most common pathogen causing cellulitis is β-hemolytic *Streptococcus* followed by *S aureus*.[5] Data from the SENTRY Antimicrobial Surveillance Program identified *S aureus* as the most common skin and soft tissue infection among complicated and hospitalized patients followed by multiple other bacteria, including *Streptococcus*.[6] However, streptococcal infections are probably under-represented in the data on infections. The under-representation is secondary to most infections being mild and not requiring patients to be hospitalized[6]; also, the true incidence is difficult to assess because of a lack of specimens and studies using unconventional identification methods.[7] *S aureus* is the most common pathogen in skin abscesses.[5] This includes community-associated methicillin-resistant *Staphylococcus aureus* (CA-MRSA), which has been seen frequently in young, healthy people and

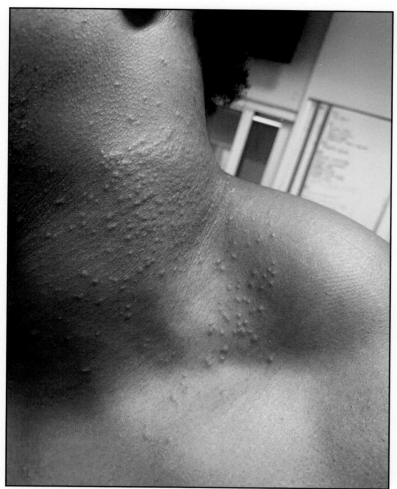

Figure 7-1. Folliculitis on the neck.

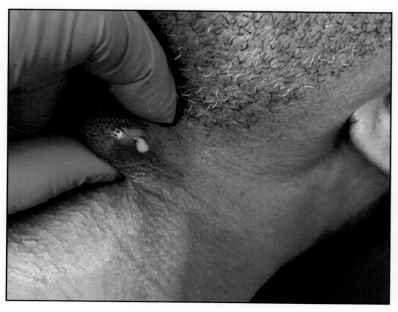

Figure 7-2. An abscess on the chin.

Figure 7-3. Impetigo.

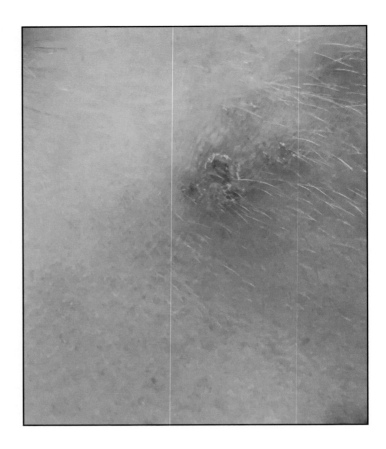

Figure 7-4. Cellulitis on the dorsal hand. Note the markings to monitor the progression of erythema.

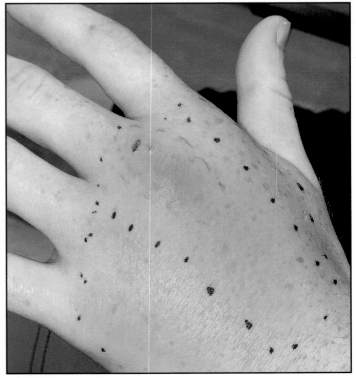

athletes at greater risk because of the close contact settings.[5,8] CA-MRSA has made treatment and cure of skin and soft tissue infections more difficult.[1] Several reasons include the resistance to commonly used antibiotics and possible increased virulence allowing infection to progress and spread more easily.[1]

Acute skin trauma provides a portal for possible infection. Although many wounds are superficial-thickness injuries that typically heal uneventfully over several weeks, they can be serious if a larger surface area is damaged or they contain foreign bodies. Acute skin trauma should initially have bleeding controlled to minimize infection risk and scarring.[9] Clinicians should assess the wound for foreign bodies, which should be removed through cleansing and debridement. Acute wounds should be cleansed with normal saline or potable tap water; there have been no differences in the rates of infection and healing between the solutions.[10] Antiseptics have been used for wound cleansing and remain an area of controversy based on possible cytotoxicity to tissues.[11]

Preparation, repair, and treatment of acute skin trauma will depend on the degree of injury, location, foreign bodies, and potential contamination. If the injury were sustained on artificial turf, there would be an increased risk of staphylococcal infection with abrasions.[12] There are different options for the closure of lacerations, which may depend on the location, depth, shape, and skin tension. For lacerations with clean straight edges and low tension, wound closure strips are a quick and easy option with low infection rates.[9] Dermal adhesives are another option for lacerations but may be a suboptimal choice for athletes because adhesives should remain dry and are not appropriate for use over areas of high skin tension.[9] There may be a risk of dehiscence because dermal adhesives have less bonding strength compared with sutures for the first 5 days of healing. Additionally, excessive moisture from perspiration can weaken the bond.[9] Wound dehiscence can delay healing and increase the risk of infection or scarring.

Clinical Features of Infected Wounds

Clinicians should monitor acute wounds for signs or symptoms of infection, and any concerns should be addressed promptly. Wound dehiscence and delayed healing may be a sign of infection. As the infection progresses, erythema, edema, warmth, and increasing pain and fever can be present. Increasing severity of infection may present with vesicles, bullae necrosis, ascending **lymphangitis**, and regional lymphadenopathy.[2] **Induration** and **fluctuance** will be present with the development of an abscess.

Treatment

Infected wounds may require treatment with topical or oral antibiotics based on the type and severity of the infection. Impetigo and simple folliculitis are treated with topical antibiotics. Deep or spreading infections along tissue planes usually require oral antibiotics. Systemic antibiotics should be used to treat cellulitis, although multiple different treatment regimens have been used.[4] For nonpurulent uncomplicated cellulitis, treatment should be directed toward β-hemolytic *Streptococcus* and methicillin-sensitive *S aureus*. Coverage should be expanded for CA-MRSA if signs and symptoms are worsening, risk factors for CA-MRSA are present, or the development of an abscess occurs.[2,4] For purulent infections such as a furuncle, a carbuncle, or an abscess, antibiotic treatment should be directed toward CA-MRSA.[3] The lesions may present as a small pustule or give the false impression of an insect or spider bite. When suspected, the patient should be removed from team activities and referred to a physician for evaluation, incision, and drainage. A tissue or drainage sample is taken for culture, and appropriate antibiotic treatment is given based on local resistance rates.[8] For a simple abscess without associated cellulitis, incision and drainage may be the only treatment necessary.[2]

Figure 7-5. An animal bite on the right hand.

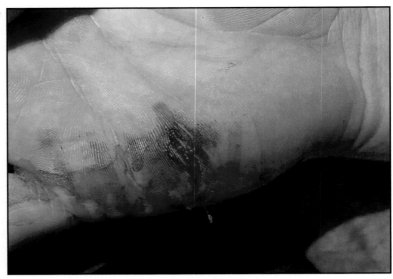

Prevention

Although most acute skin trauma can be managed during athletic, recreational, and work activities with proper interventions and a return to play or work, clinicians should reassess the patient and wound thoroughly afterward. Wounds should undergo appropriate cleansing, debridement, and dressing interventions to optimize wound healing and prevent infection. There is good evidence that meticulous wound cleansing is associated with reduced rates of infection.[13] The use of occlusive dressings also contributes to lower rates of infection, higher rates of healing, and lower levels of pain.[14] Topical and oral antimicrobials may also play a role in the prevention of infection. Prophylactic oral antibiotics are rarely required for acute skin trauma. Wounds that are not grossly contaminated and have received appropriate cleansing and debridement have very low overall infection rates.[2] The routine use of antibiotics has not demonstrated a benefit in reducing the rates of infection, although investigations have typically excluded participants who may have been at higher risk.[14] Antibiotic prophylaxis should be considered with contaminated wounds; deep puncture wounds; wounds involving the tendon, bone, or joint; lower extremity wounds; larger wounds or wounds with jagged edges; the presence of a foreign body; or immunosuppressed patients.[11,14] Prophylactic oral antibiotics are also advisable for a patient who has a wound secondary to the mouth or a human or animal bite (Figure 7-5). These wounds may contain bacteria from the oral flora of the biter, the skin of the victim, and the environment.[15] *Streptococcus pyogenes* and anaerobic bacteria may be present in human bites. Teeth can lodge bacteria into a deeper laceration with signs of infection possibly starting as early as 24 hours after the bite.[15]

Topical antibiotics may be preferable over oral antibiotics because they result in a higher concentration at the wound site with lower systemic side effects and incidence of antimicrobial resistance.[16] There is limited evidence to support the use of topical antibiotics in uncomplicated minor wounds to prevent infection. However, 2 randomized controlled trials demonstrated a reduction in the rates of infection with the use of topical antibiotics among traumatic wounds.[17,18] Therefore, topical antibiotics for infection prophylaxis in minor, uncomplicated soft tissue wounds should be considered. A variety of topical antibiotics are often used in double or triple combinations to extend the spectrum of coverage and decrease resistance. Neomycin is active against staphylococci and most aerobic gram-negative bacteria; however, streptococci and gram-positive bacilli are resistant. Neomycin has a higher prevalence of skin sensitivity; rashes form in 6% to 8% of patients, and allergic contact dermatitis is the most common adverse effect. Neomycin also has the potential for systemic toxicity, including hearing loss.[16,17] Bacitracin is active against gram-positive organisms, including *S aureus* and *streptococcus pyogenes*; other β-hemolytic streptococci and gram-negative bacteria are resistant.[17] There is potential for burning, itching, or irritation at the site with the use of bacitracin. Allergic contact reactions can occur and be delayed 96 hours. Rare cases of anaphylactic reactions have also been reported with bacitracin.[16] Polymyxin B is active only against gram-negative bacteria. Given its limited activity against gram-positive bacteria, polymyxin B should be used in combination with other topical antimicrobials.[17] Mupirocin has been mainly used to prevent and treat a staphylococcal infection. Widespread use of mupirocin can lead to resistance, and there is potential for cytotoxicity and delayed healing. Allergic contact dermatitis can occur, and systemic absorption could lead to renal toxicity.[16,17]

Skin antiseptics can decrease bacterial counts and the number of bacteria colonizing the skin. Antiseptics may have toxic effects when used directly on the wound bed and should be used with caution. However, antiseptics can safely be used on the periwound tissue. Topical antiseptics include chlorhexidine, povidone-iodine, and isopropyl alcohol. Chlorhexidine is most active against gram-positive bacteria, with some activity against gram-negative bacteria. It is considered an extremely safe topical agent with only mild adverse effects, such as skin irritation.[17] Povidone-iodine has the broadest spectrum of activity and produces antimicrobial effects by releasing free iodine. However, allergic reactions are possible, and systemic absorption may influence thyroid function or affect renal function.[16,17] Isopropyl alcohol is bactericidal and exhibits a broad spectrum of antimicrobial activity, which is best achieved at a concentration of 60% to 90%.[17] Antiseptics are effective at reducing surgical site infections, with chlorhexidine or a combination of chlorhexidine and isopropyl alcohol being more effective than iodine.[19] Therefore, skin antisepsis may be beneficial in cleansing the periwound tissue before the closure of traumatic incisions and lacerations with wound closure strips or dermal adhesives.[2]

The rates of infection among traumatic lacerations and postoperative incisions can be influenced by the time from injury to treatment and exposure to water or showering. As time elapses from injury to treatment, bacteria colonize and multiply in a wound. In wounds containing $> 10^5$ organisms per gram of tissue, more than 50% of patients will develop an infection. The mean time to reach $> 10^5$ organisms per gram of tissue is 5.17 hours.[2] To reduce the rates of infection, some suggest the closure of lacerations within 6 hours; others recommend anywhere from 3 to 24 hours.[13] There is a lack of evidence to support a specific cutoff time for the closure of lacerations. Many studies contained patients prescribed antibiotics for older wounds, which may have confounded the results.[13] After the closure of lacerations and incisions, there is a concern that water exposure or showering affects wound healing and the risk for infection. Among postoperative incisions, the patient is often allowed to shower at 48 hours when re-epithelialization has occurred. Although there is limited evidence on postoperative showering and the rates of infection and healing, an evidence-based review found no differences in the rates of infection between showering within the first 48 hours and after 3 days.[20]

ADVERSE REACTIONS

Adverse reactions may occur with materials used in the acute skin trauma management plan. Reactions can range from a simple rash to a serious, life-threatening event. Allergic contact dermatitis may occur with many products, including antiseptics, antimicrobials, adhesives, and dressings.[2,16,17,21,22] Allergic contact dermatitis is an immune-mediated type IV delayed hypersensitivity reaction. It typically presents 48 hours after exposure at the site of skin contact.[23] Neomycin and bacitracin are 2 common topical antibiotic allergens.[21,23] Although the incidence is low, allergic contact dermatitis should be suspected with the development of **pruritic**, erythematous, and edematous papules or vesicles.[21] Although treated similarly, irritant contact dermatitis is distinguished from allergic contact dermatitis by the presentation of well-defined erythematous patches or plaques

Figure 7-6. Irritant contact dermatitis on the lateral elbow.

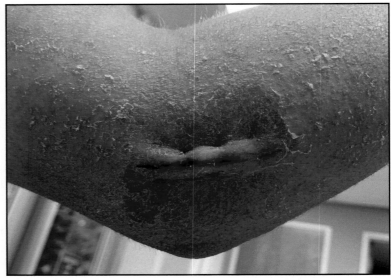

(Figure 7-6). Irritant contact dermatitis may also have vesicles or bullae.[22,23] Irritant contact dermatitis is not immune-mediated, and a rash develops rapidly and sometimes within minutes of contact.[23] It is more critical to distinguish irritant and allergic contact dermatitis rashes from developing cellulitis.[22] For the treatment of allergic and irritant contact dermatitis, the offending substance should be removed and topical corticosteroids applied to the area. More severe cases require the use of oral steroids and antihistamines.[2] Anaphylaxis can rarely occur with contact allergens. This reaction has been reported with the use of bacitracin and chlorhexidine.[24,25] Anaphylaxis is an immunoglobulin E–mediated allergic reaction presenting quickly with **urticaria** (Figure 7-7), dyspnea, nausea, vomiting, diarrhea, and dizziness. Anaphylaxis is emergent and can be fatal. Treatment includes immediate epinephrine, antihistamines, oxygen, intravenous fluids, and possibly corticosteroids.[24,25] Antiseptics such as povidone-iodine and chlorhexidine have been associated with chemical burns.[26-28] Burns can occur with prolonged contact or pooling of the antiseptic or with an occlusive device or dressing. Chemical burns are typically painful and have well-demarcated erythema, vesicles, and bullae. Simple burns can be treated with topical antibiotics and dressings that promote healing.[28] If the burn is more severe, a referral for specialty care should be made.

Nonocclusive and occlusive dressings used for acute wounds can also result in adverse reactions. Allergic and irritant contact dermatitis have been associated with hydrocolloids and adhesives related to the dressings.[29,30] Allergic and irritant contact dermatitis have also been caused by adhesives (eg, cyanoacrylate and benzoin) used to close lacerations.[22] Occlusive dressings can also cause folliculitis.[31] Folliculitis is an infection of the hair follicles and presents with erythematous papules and pustules in the periwound tissue (see Figure 7-1). Removal of the dressing and topical antibiotics may be an adequate treatment for most patients. Referral and oral antibiotics should be considered when clinical features are not resolving over the next 48 to 72 hours or with the development of additional lesions.[32] Maceration of the periwound tissue can result from dressings and contribute to patient discomfort and delayed healing (Figure 7-8).[33] Excessive moisture produced by perspiration, wound exudate, and dressing failure can soften and break down the periwound tissue. Maceration is identified by white discoloration of the periwound tissue.[33] Red discoloration and inflammation of the periwound tissue accompanied with burning, itching, and stinging can be associated with erythematous maceration.[34] Wounds with maceration require dressing removal, reassessment, and revisions to the management plan.[2] Adverse reactions can occur secondary to the closure of lacerations and incisions with dermal adhesives and sutures. Although dermal adhesives provide the advantages of ease of use for the clinician and comfort for the patient, adhesives can

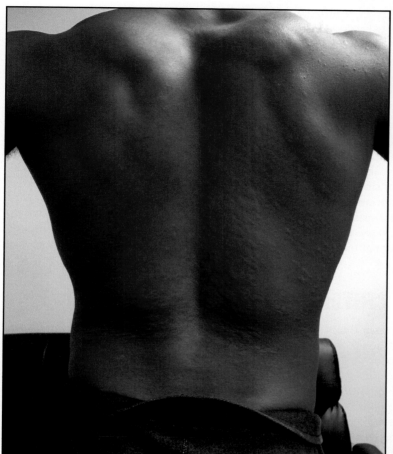

Figure 7-7. Urticaria on the back.

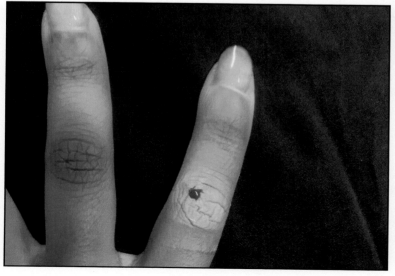

Figure 7-8. Maceration on the dorsal second finger caused by an adhesive gauze strip.

produce foreign body reactions.[35] Clinically, these reactions present as tenderness over the wound site followed by the development of a mass.[35] Wound dehiscence can occur with dermal adhesives in areas around a joint or high skin tension or with the early removal of sutures. Dehiscence can result in poor wound healing and increase the risk of infection. Sutures left in place beyond recommended durations can produce scarring at the wound site. Generally, sutures should be removed from the face after 3 to 5 days and from the hands, feet, back, and over joints or areas of high tension after 10 to 14 days; otherwise, they should be removed after 7 to 10 days.[11,14]

Underlying health conditions of the patient obtained through an assessment need to be considered because comorbid illnesses and conditions, current medications, and lifestyle can affect interventions and healing outcomes.[2] Diabetes can increase the risk of delayed wound healing and susceptibility to infection. Other diseases that may impair wound healing include chronic renal insufficiency, acute or chronic liver disease, peripheral vascular disease, cancer, or AIDS.[36,37] Medications that patients are taking can also impair wound healing. Topical and systemic steroids,[38] nonsteroidal anti-inflammatories,[37,38] anticoagulants,[37,38] antimicrobials,[38] vasodilators,[39] antihistamines,[39] antiplatelets,[39] vasoconstrictors,[38] and chemotherapeutic agents[37] may delay healing. Smoking and alcohol consumption may suppress wound healing due to multifactorial reasons.[39]

CRITERIA FOR REFERRAL

The majority of acute skin trauma can be managed in athletic training or similar health care facilities without complications.[2] Deep wounds that require advanced closure with sutures or staples, wounds with nerve or tendon damage that may require surgical intervention, and wounds with heavy contamination that require advanced cleansing and debridement and possible antibiotic prophylaxis require physician referral. Physician referral should be considered for patients who are immunocompromised or have underlying medical problems such as diabetes, chronic kidney disease, chronic liver disease, or AIDS, which are associated with increased risks of delayed healing and infection. Uncomplicated acute wounds being managed and reassessed daily require physician referral with the development of clinical features of infection. The triggers for referral include wound dehiscence; delay in normal healing; spread of erythema from the wound; development of warmth in the periwound tissue; purulent discharge; development of pustules, induration, or fluctuance; and pain out of proportion to the injury. Despite initial interventions, patients with worsening symptoms of adverse reactions require referral for further assessment. Clinicians should also refer patients for the development of signs and symptoms with unclear etiology or potential association with infection. Although rare, anaphylaxis can occur and requires activation of the emergency action plan and referral. Anaphylaxis may be more likely if there has been a prior skin reaction to a product causing sensitization.

SUMMARY

Acute skin trauma is common in athletic, recreational, and work activities. Proper management with daily monitoring and reassessments can produce optimal healing and function and lessen the risk of adverse outcomes. Secondary purulent and nonpurulent infections may occur after injury. Prompt recognition and referral for evaluation and treatment can prevent the progression of the infection. Appropriate cleansing, debridement, and dressing interventions and antimicrobials for patients with risk factors play a critical role in preventing infection. Clinicians should recognize patient health status and reactions to the cleansing, debridement, and dressing interventions and materials used to manage acute skin trauma for the development of adverse reactions. Timely assessment allows for proper treatment of the reaction and a reduction in harm to the patient. The recognition of when patients should be referred is essential in the management of potential infections and adverse reactions. Clinicians should immediately address any concerns and refer patients for further assessment when necessary. Developing the basic knowledge of skin and soft tissue infections and the potential adverse effects of interventions regarding recognition and response will improve overall patient care.

REFERENCES

1. Mitchell JJ, Jackson JM, Anwar A, Singleton SB. Bacterial sport-related skin and soft-tissue infections (SSTIs): An ongoing problem among a diverse range of athletes. *JBJS Rev.* 2017;5(1):e4.

2. Beam JW, Buckley B, Holcomb WR, Ciocca M. National Athletic Trainers' Association position statement: Management of acute skin trauma. *J Athl Train.* 2016;51(12):1053-1070.

3. Bystritsky R, Chambers H. Cellulitis and soft tissue infections. *Ann Intern Med.* 2018;168(3):ITC17-ITC32.

4. Raff AB, Kroshinsky D. Cellulitis: A review. *JAMA.* 2016;316(3):325-337.

5. Poulakou G, Lagou S, Tsiodras S. What's new in the epidemiology of skin and soft tissue infections in 2018? *Curr Opin Infect Dis.* 2019;32(2):77-86.

6. Moet GJ, Jones RN, Biedenbach DJ, Stilwell MG, Fritsche TR. Contemporary causes of skin and soft tissue infections in North America, Latin America, and Europe: Report from the SENTRY Antimicrobial Surveillance Program (1998-2004). *Diagn Microbiol Infect Dis.* 2007;57(1):7-13.

7. Rajan S. Skin and soft-tissue infections: Classifying and treating a spectrum. *Cleve Clin J Med.* 2012;79(1):57-66.

8. Zinder SM, Basler RSW, Foley J, Scarlata C, Vasily DB. National Athletic Trainers' Association position statement: Skin diseases. *J Athl Train.* 2010;45(4):411-428.

9. Ediger MJ. Closure options for skin lacerations. *Int J Athl Ther Train.* 2010;15(2):19-22.

10. Beam JW. Wound cleansing: Water or saline? *J Athl Train.* 2006;41(2):196-197.

11. Honsik KA, Romeo MW, Hawley CJ, Romeo SJ, Romeo JP. Sideline skin and wound care for acute injuries. *Curr Sports Med Rep.* 2007;6(3):147-154.

12. Twomey DM, Petrass LA, Fleming P, Lenehan K. Abrasion injuries on artificial turf: A systematic review. *J Sci Med Sport.* 2019;22(5):550-556.

13. Zehtabchi S, Tan A, Yadav K, Badawy A, Lucchesi M. The impact of wound age on the infection rate of simple lacerations repaired in the emergency department. *Injury.* 2012;43(11):1793-1798.

14. Mankowitz SL. Laceration management. *J Emerg Med.* 2017;53(3):369-382.

15. Brook I. Management of human and animal bite wound infection: An overview. *Curr Infect Dis Rep.* 2009;11(5):389-395.

16. Punjataewakupt A, Napavichayanun S, Aramwit P. The downside of antimicrobial agents for wound healing. *Eur J Clin Microbiol Infect Dis.* 2019;38(1):39-54.

17. Williamson DA, Carter GP, Howden BP. Current and emerging topical antibacterials and antiseptics: Agents, action, and resistance patterns. *Clin Microbiol Rev.* 2017;30(3):827-860.

18. Waterbrook AL, Hiller K, Hays DP, Berkman M. Do topical antibiotics help prevent infection in minor traumatic uncomplicated soft tissue wounds? *Ann Emerg Med.* 2013;61(1):86-88.

19. Lee I, Agarwal RK, Lee BY, Fishman NO, Umscheid CA. Systematic review and cost analysis comparing use of chlorhexidine with use of iodine for preoperative skin antisepsis to prevent surgical site infection. *Infect Control Hosp Epidemiol.* 2010;31(12):1219-1229. doi:10.1086/657134

20. Copeland-Halperin LR, Reategui Via y Rada ML, Levy J, Shank N, Funderburk CD, Shin JH. Does the timing of postoperative showering impact infection rates? A systematic review and meta-analysis. *J Plast Reconstr Aesthet Surg.* 2020;73(7):1306-1311.

21. Bonamonte D, De Marco A, Giuffrida R, et al. Topical antibiotics in the dermatological clinical practice: Indications, efficacy, and adverse effects. *Dermatol Ther.* 2020;33(6):e13824. doi:10.1111/dth.13824

22. Thornton NJ, Gibson BR, Ferry AM. Contact dermatitis and medical adhesives: A review. *Cureus.* 2021;13(3):e14090. doi:10.7759/cureus.14090

23. Nguyen HL, Yiannias JA. Contact dermatitis to medications and skin products. *Clin Rev Allergy Immunol.* 2019;56(1):41-59.

24. Saryan JA, Dammin TC, Bouras AE. Anaphylaxis to topical bacitracin zinc ointment. *Am J Emerg Med.* 1998;16(5):512-513.

25. Krautheim AB, Jermann THM, Bircher AJ. Chlorhexidine anaphylaxis: Case report and review of the literature. *Contact Dermatitis.* 2004;50(3):113-116.

26. Lowe DO, Knowles SR, Weber EA, Railton CJ, Shear NH. Povidone-iodine-induced burn: Case report and review of the literature. *Pharmacotherapy.* 2006;26(11):1641-1645.

27. Sanders TH, Hawken SM. Chlorhexidine burns after shoulder arthroscopy. *Am J Orthop (Belle Mead NJ).* 2012;41(4):172-174.

28. Rees A, Sherrod Q, Young L. Chemical burn from povidone-iodine: Case and review. *J Drugs Dermatol.* 2011;10(4):414-417.

29. Suhng EA, Byun JY, Choi YW, Myung KB, Choi HY. A case of allergic contact dermatitis due to DuoDERM Extrathin. *Ann Dermatol.* 2011;23(suppl 3):S387-S389.

30. Mestach L, Huygens S, Goossens A, Gilissen L. Allergic contact dermatitis caused by acrylic-based medical dressings and adhesives. *Contact Dermatitis.* 2018;79(2):81-84.

31. Zhao H, He Y, Wei Q, Ying Y. Medical adhesive-related skin injury prevalence at the peripherally inserted central catheter insertion site: A cross-sectional, multiple-center study. *J Wound Ostomy Continence Nurs.* 2018;45(1):22-25.

32. Nowicka D, Baglaj-Oleszczuk M, Maj J. Infectious diseases of the skin in contact sports. *Adv Clin Exp Med.* 2020;29(12):1491-1495.

33. Whitehead F, Giampieri S, Graham T, Grocott P. Identifying, managing and preventing skin maceration: A rapid review of the clinical evidence. *J Wound Care.* 2017;26(4):159-165.

34. Hollinworth H. Challenges in protecting peri-wound skin. *Nurs Stand.* 2009;24(7):53-54, 56, 58.

35. Dragu A, Unglaub F, Schwarz S, et al. Foreign body reaction after usage of tissue adhesives for skin closure: A case report and review of the literature. *Arch Orthop Trauma Surg.* 2009;129(2):167-169.

36. Khalil H, Cullen M, Chambers H, Carroll M, Walker J. Elements affecting wound healing time: An evidence based analysis. *Wound Repair Regen.* 2015;23(4):550-556.

37. Khalil H, Cullen M, Chambers H, McGrail M. Medications affecting healing: An evidence-based analysis. *Int Wound J.* 2017;14(6):1340-1345.

38. Beitz JM. Pharmacologic impact (aka "breaking bad") of medications on wound healing and wound development: A literature-based overview. *Ostomy Wound Manage.* 2017;63(3):18-35.

39. Wigston C, Hassan S, Turvey S, et al. Impact of medications and lifestyle factors on wound healing: A pilot study. *Wounds UK.* 2013;9(1):22-28.

8

CLINICAL PRACTICE SCENARIOS

Clinicians will frequently encounter acute skin trauma, and appropriate management of the patient and wound is critical to promote healing and lessen the risk of adverse reactions. The chapters in this book focus on individual components of wound management, such as the assessment and diagnosis process, cleansing, debridement, dressing interventions and procedures, etiology and identification of infection and adverse outcomes, patient monitoring and education, and management environment and infection control. Successful management of acute skin trauma requires clinicians to think beyond individual components; management includes evaluating the patient and considering wound, clinician, and environmental factors simultaneously to develop, implement, and monitor the management plan and patient.

This chapter links the individual components and factors together to assist clinicians in developing appropriate management plans and necessary revisions to the plans as warranted. The scenarios may present patient history, assessment findings, diagnosis, initial management plan, reassessment findings, or unique situations among various clinical settings. Clinicians can work through

DOI: 10.1201/9781003523055-8

each case and consider appropriate interventions and actions based on the information provided. The author's recommendations and solutions follow each scenario. The Things to Consider sections provide information clinicians should weigh and evaluate in the clinical decision-making process for each scenario. Clinicians can refer to individual chapters to answer questions or find further explanations for the recommendations.

SCENARIO 1

Preseason practices for football, soccer, and volleyball teams are underway, and athletes report to the athletic training facility with abrasions, blisters, and lacerations of various etiologies and characteristics. The athletic training staff completes assessments for each athlete and begins to design individual management plans. The plans include cleansing and debridement of the skin trauma with normal saline or potable tap water irrigation. However, product shortages and supply chain issues have delayed the purchasing process, specifically the delivery of wound care supplies, including syringes and plastic cannulas, for this fiscal year. Based on this information, what actions are appropriate in this situation?

Recommendations

Several alternatives are available for using 35-mL syringes and 18- to 20-gauge plastic cannulas for irrigation. Normal and sterile saline can be delivered to the wound bed and periwound tissue through pressurized canisters, squeeze bottles, bulb syringes, and trigger spray devices. The canisters and bottles can be purchased with various amounts of solution and sprayed or poured onto the tissue. Many of the trigger spray devices are attached to saline bottles for use. Potable tap water in unopened bottled water, clean sports squeeze water bottles, and bulb syringes can be used for cleansing and debridement. Bottled and sports squeeze water bottles can be opened and poured onto the tissue. Clinicians can cut a small hole in the bottled water's cap or use the sports bottle valve to increase irrigation pressures. Bulb syringes are first loaded with saline or tap water and are available in manual squeeze and spray designs. Showering is safe with postoperative incisions and can be used for larger traumatic wounds. If the size of the body area and wound allow, tap water rinses from a sink faucet can also be used for cleansing. Normal saline and potable tap water should be delivered to the wound bed between 98.6°F and 107.6°F (37°C and 42°C).

Things to Consider

Evidence-based guidelines recommend irrigation for the cleansing of acute skin trauma to create an environment conducive to healing. Normal saline or potable tap water should be delivered to the wound bed at pressures between 4 and 15 pounds per square inch (psi; 27.58-103.42 kPa). A 35-mL syringe and an 18- to 20-gauge needle hub or plastic cannula will deliver solutions at 7 to 11 psi (48.26-75.84 kPa). In the absence of syringes, hubs, or cannulas, clinicians must consider the benefits and limitations of alternative irrigation techniques before use with patients. Good evidence supports the use of normal saline and potable tap water for wound cleansing. Water from a faucet should be from a treated supply and run a few minutes before use with a wound. Pressurized canisters, squeeze bottles, bulb syringes, bottled water, sports bottles, showering, and faucet rinses are appropriate as irrigation alternatives to deliver normal saline and tap water to the wound bed and periwound tissue. However, the pressure of the solutions delivered with these techniques cannot be controlled and may not be in the recommended range of 4 to 15 psi. Several trigger spray designs deliver normal saline in the recommended psi range and are available with guards to reduce splash back. Despite the lower pressure limitation, the use of normal saline or potable tap water is safe and nontoxic to tissues compared with the use of topical antiseptics. Additionally, irrigation through these alternative methods reduces the risk of disrupting the moisture balance of the wound bed, macerating the periwound tissue, mechanically damaging the granulation tissue, and introducing microorganisms to the tissues that can occur with hydrotherapy and scrubbing and swabbing cleansing techniques. Lastly, if resources prohibit the purchase of saline, the solution can be made in a facility for a minimal cost. Make the solution by first obtaining a clean container and spoon. Pour 1 qt (0.95 L) distilled water or 1 qt (0.95 L) tap water that has been boiled for 5 minutes into the container. Add 2 teaspoons (9.86 mL) table salt to the water and mix the solution until the salt is completely dissolved. Do not use the boiled solution until cooled between 98.6°F and 107.6°F (37°C and 42°C). Store the solution in a tightly closed glass or plastic container and use it with an irrigation technique within 1 week.

SCENARIO 2

A high school basketball athlete sustains a superficial-thickness lateral forearm laceration during practice. An assessment, irrigation with tap water, and the application of premoistened woven sterile gauze and self-adherent wrap dressings allow a return to practice. After practice, the dressings are removed, and a reassessment is performed. The wound is irrigated, and a primary film dressing and secondary adhesive gauze strips on the dressing edges are applied. The patient leaves for home and is instructed to return the following morning for reassessment. The patient presents with the primary and secondary dressings removed the next day. The patient reports that his parents removed the dressings, fearing the brownish fluid visible under the dressing over the wound. Based on the information, what actions are appropriate in this situation?

Recommendations

Reassess the patient, wound bed, and periwound tissue. The findings may reveal contamination and dehydration of the wound bed tissues based on the removal of the dressing and exposure of the wound to the external environment. With no clinical features of adverse reactions, cleanse the wound with normal saline or tap water irrigation and debride, if necessary, with an atraumatic technique. Based on the assessment findings, choose and apply a dressing that promotes moisture retention. Promote cooperation and adherence to the management plan by educating the patient on the goals and guidelines of the plan, home care, and self-monitoring. Because the patient lives with family, education of the family will also be required to achieve intervention and healing outcomes.

Things to Consider

Patient education is paramount to the successful management of acute skin trauma. In this situation, family education is also necessary. Advancements in acute wound care have drastically changed what and why interventions are used. Perhaps the most significant changes have occurred with occlusive dressings and the creation of a moist wound environment. Many patients lack the knowledge and experience with modern dressings and the concept of moist wound healing and believe drying of the wound and the formation of eschar promote healing. Clear communication and education will provide the patient and family with the knowledge, explanations, and rationale for understanding and adherence to the management plan. Clinicians can use published position statements and clinical guidelines to develop educational materials to supplement education efforts.

SCENARIO 3

During practice, an intercollegiate softball athlete performs base running drills and slides into third base on a hard, clay infield. The shear force tears the pant leg and produces trauma to the lateral proximal thigh. The patient is initially evaluated and treated on the field and immediately taken to the athletic training facility for further assessment. The assessment reveals a full-thickness lateral, proximal thigh abrasion. Past medical history is unremarkable. The patient showers in the locker room and returns to the athletic training facility. The wound is cleansed and debrided with normal saline irrigation to remove the remaining clay pieces. The depth of tissue damage and the production of heavy exudate will necessitate several dressing transitions in the management plan throughout the healing process. The clinician begins to consider dressing selection and transitions for the patient and full-thickness abrasion. Based on this information, what actions are appropriate in this situation?

Recommendations

Initially, high-absorbent alginate and high-absorbent and moderate to high moisture vapor transmission rate foam dressings are indicated to provide occlusion, create a moist wound environment, and manage the heavy exudate produced by the full-thickness abrasion. A secondary film dressing can be used to secure these dressings to the periwound tissue. As normal healing progresses, re-epithelization, the formation of a new extracellular matrix, and a decrease in exudate production occur. These changes require transitioning to less absorbent dressings to promote an optimal wound environment. Alginates, foams, and hydrocolloids are recommended as primary dressings for moderate to heavy exudate levels, and a film secondary dressing may be needed. Exudate levels will continue to decrease during healing, and transitions to hydrocolloid and hydrogel dressings are indicated with minimal to moderate exudate amounts over the wound. During the last stage of healing and minimal levels of exudate, film and hydrogel dressings are warranted to trap or donate moisture to the wound bed. Nonocclusive woven or nonwoven sterile gauze, nonadherent pads, or adhesive strips and patches can be considered alternative dressings in the management plan. Complete healing, demonstrated by a pale pink color of the wound bed and full wound contraction and resurfacing, signals cessation of dressing wear.

Things to Consider

Dressing selection and transitions are based on patient, wound, and dressing factors. They should correspond with the cellular and chemical changes in the wound bed during the normal progression of healing. A critical factor in dressing transitions is the level of exudate production. The heavy exudate associated with the full-thickness abrasion excluded many dressings from the selection process; few dressings possess the ability to manage heavy amounts of exudate and promote a moist wound environment. With the progression of healing and the decrease in exudate levels, the continued use of high-absorbent dressings can desiccate the wound bed, adhere the dressing to the wound bed, and delay healing. Dressing transitions should complement cellular and chemical changes in the wound bed to manage and remove excess exudate or donate moisture to the wound to create a moist healing environment. Occlusive dressings are recommended to interact with the wound, promote healing, and lessen the risk of infection. These dressings are constructed with materials to manage varying exudate levels and can remain on the wound bed for longer periods than nonocclusive dressings. However, dressing changes and reassessment of the management plan are required with dressing saturation and integrity or barrier issues. In the absence of occlusive dressings, nonocclusive dressings can be used. Transitions are not required with nonocclusive dressings.

However, daily changes are required to lessen the risk of periwound tissue maceration; dressing leakage; strike-through; and desiccation, infection, and delayed healing. Normal wound healing is an orderly process of 3 phases with overlapping activities and events. The consequences of inappropriate dressing selection and transitions can result in adverse patient and healing outcomes. However, daily monitoring and reassessments and competence with wound healing and the management plan can identify patient and wound characteristics and the effectiveness of interventions to guide dressing transitions.

SCENARIO 4

A patient is assessed and diagnosed with a partial-thickness lateral, proximal lower leg abrasion. Past medical history is unremarkable. The management plan includes the application of a hydrocolloid primary dressing and an adhesive gauze secondary dressing. The patient is reassessed the following day, and no changes are reported. The patient is not seen for several days. On postinjury day 4, the patient presents with redness and inflammation of the periwound tissue and reports burning and stinging sensations in the tissues under the dressing. Inspection reveals swelling of the dressing over the wound extending to the dressing edges, separation of the dressing edges from the periwound tissue, and moderate leakage of wound exudate and dressing gel. Based on the information, what actions are appropriate in this situation?

Recommendations

The clinical features likely indicate the development of erythematous maceration of the periwound tissue. Erythematous maceration is caused by the production of heavy exudate, the inability of the dressing to manage exudate over the wound, or prolonged dressing wear. Remove the primary and secondary dressings and irrigate the wound bed and periwound tissue with normal saline. Cover the wound with woven or nonwoven sterile gauze lightly premoistened with normal saline and immediately refer the patient for further assessment. Infection can contribute to the production of heavy exudate. After referral and diagnosis, reassess the dressing selection in the management plan. The short-term goal is management of the heavy exudate. Woven and nonwoven gauze or nonadhesive foams or alginates can be used as primary dressings. A nonadhesive secondary dressing, such as sterile roll gauze or nonadherent tapes and wraps, can protect the periwound tissue from further trauma.

Things to Consider

Based on the initial assessment and diagnosis, the selection of a hydrocolloid was appropriate. The patient's medical history was absent of comorbid conditions, allergies to dressing materials, current medications, and past complications with healing. Partial-thickness wounds typically produce moderate levels of exudate, and hydrocolloids, hydrogels, alginates, foams, woven and nonwoven sterile gauze, and adhesive strips and patches can be considered. The reassessment on postinjury day 1 was normal, with the dressing intact and no clinical features of adverse reactions. However, the patient was not seen again until day 4. During this period, the hydrocolloid was unable to manage the heavy exudate, allowing the exudate to hyperhydrate the periwound tissue and compromise the barrier properties of the dressing. The clinical features of erythematous maceration and signs of dressing failure may have been observed before postinjury day 4, allowing an earlier referral and lower risk of delayed healing. This situation highlights the importance of daily patient reassessments to evaluate the effectiveness of interventions and patient responses.

SCENARIO 5

An intercollegiate swimmer participates in a 5K charity run over the weekend and suffers a plantar foot blister. An assessment the following day in the athletic training facility reveals an open, partial-thickness blister. The assessment is otherwise unremarkable. The wound is cleansed, debrided, and prepared for dressing application and a planned return to aquatic activities. Based on the information, what actions are appropriate in this situation?

Recommendations

The selection of a dressing is based on the characteristics of the wound; the types and availability of dressings; and the health, needs, and activity level of the patient. Several nonocclusive and occlusive dressings are indicated for secondary closure of partial-thickness wounds. Based on the plantar foot location, the dressing must protect the wound from shear, friction, and pressure and maintain integrity, physical properties, and adherence to the periwound tissue during ambulation. The return to aquatic activities will require the application of a waterproof, impermeable dressing that will maintain occlusion throughout the activity. Based on these factors, a hydrogel or hydrocolloid primary dressing is recommended to protect the granulation tissue and promote a moist healing environment. A secondary film dressing with waterproof and impermeable properties is required with the hydrogel and hydrocolloid to adhere the primary dressing and provide occlusion. Daily, or more frequent, reassessment of the patient and the wound must be performed with careful inspection of the film dressing to identify integrity and barrier concerns. Evidence of wrinkling or bunching and the formation of channels in the dressing, separation of the dressing edges from the periwound tissue, excessive accumulation of moisture or exudate under the dressing, or leakage warrant an immediate dressing change. Additional dressing changes may be experienced based on exposure to aquatic activities.

Things to Consider

The return to aquatic activities can increase the risk of infection and cross-contamination from the water, and dressing selection is critical to prevent adverse reactions and promote healing. Woven and nonwoven sterile gauze, nonadherent pads, adhesive strips and patches, alginate, and foam dressings can be used with partial-thickness wounds with moderate exudate. However, these dressings lack the thickness to protect the wound from shear, friction, and pressure during ambulation. The nonocclusive dressings do not promote moisture retention and provide occlusion of the wound bed. The recommended secondary film dressing must remain intact over the wound and adhere to the periwound tissue to provide impermeability and occlusion during aquatic activities. The adhesive backing of films is sufficient to maintain adherence of the dressing with bathing, showering, and physical activities that produce perspiration. However, prolonged exposure to moisture can lessen the adhesive bond, allow separation of the dressing edges from the periwound tissue, and compromise the impermeable barrier. Several additional techniques can be considered to enhance dressing adherence. Adhesive gauze strips can be applied to the edges of the secondary film dressing. Clinicians can also consider the application of a separate, waterproof film over the secondary film dressing. This separate dressing can be larger than the secondary film dressing, allowing additional adherence to the periwound tissue. Adhesive gauze strips can also be applied to the edges of the separate film. However, this dressing will likely adhere to the secondary film dressing. Upon removal, the secondary dressing can be removed and the primary dressing disrupted, causing unnecessary dressing changes and possible delayed healing. Nonadherent, self-adherent, and adherent tapes and wraps will secure the primary and secondary dressings during the activity. However, each will absorb moisture, become saturated, and loosen from the periwound tissue during aquatic activities.

SCENARIO 6

Midway through the fall intercollegiate sports season, a cluster of methicillin-resistant *Staphylococcus aureus* (MRSA) infections occur among basketball, field hockey, and soccer athletes. The cases are reported to local and state health departments, and an investigation is ongoing. The infected athletes are receiving treatment and monitoring by the medical team. Athletic training facility operations, team practices, and competitions continue, and various skin trauma occurs among noninfected athletes. The athletic training staff discusses whether changes are needed to current cleansing, debridement, and dressing interventions to lessen the risk of new cases of MRSA during the treatment of the injured athletes. Based on this information, what actions are appropriate in this situation?

Recommendations

The management plans should consist of cleansing, debridement, and dressing interventions guided by standard precautions and an established infection control plan. Cleansing of the wound bed can be performed with normal saline or tap water irrigation to remove microorganisms and foreign debris. Showering can also be considered. Whirlpool baths and soaks may increase the risk of cross-contamination and are not indicated. Scrubbing and swabbing can contaminate and damage granulation tissue and should be avoided. However, scrubbing and swabbing the periwound tissue with a topical antiseptic can lower bacterial counts. Autolytic, conservative sharp, irrigation, or wet-to-moist debridement can be used with noninfected wounds. Scrubbing, wet-to-dry, hydrotherapy, and chemical methods can damage the wound bed and increase the risk of contamination and are not recommended. Based on patient and wound characteristics and the available supplies, occlusive dressings are recommended in this situation to lessen the risk of cross-contamination and infection and promote healing. Topical antimicrobial agents can be considered in combination with occlusive dressings. Conduct daily monitoring and reassessment of the patients and the wounds to identify the effectiveness of interventions and the development of infection.

Things to Consider

The direct and indirect transmission and risk factors of compromised skin integrity and open wounds associated with MRSA warrant thorough reviews of management plans and interventions for acute skin trauma to prevent further cases. The interventions selected must promote healing and lessen the risk of infection. The recommended cleansing and debridement techniques have been shown to create an optimal healing environment and reduce infection rates among various wound types. The selection of an appropriate dressing is paramount in achieving healing outcomes. Published guidelines for managing and preventing skin infections in athletics recommend that all open wounds and noninfectious skin conditions be adequately protected and properly covered for return to participation. This recommendation suggests the wound or condition receives appropriate care in a comprehensive management plan and is covered with a dressing that can manage exudate, maintain impermeability, prevent leakage, and remain secure to the periwound tissue throughout practices and competitions. Nonocclusive dressings possess high permeability and lack barrier properties to the external environment. They have variable absorption abilities that promote desiccation of the wound bed, increase risks of cross-contamination and infection, and promote leakage. Occlusive dressings are semipermeable and impermeable, provide barrier capabilities to the inward and outward penetration of microorganisms, and manage and maintain exudate to promote a moist healing environment and lower infection rates. Occlusive dressings produce greater rates of healing than nonocclusive dressings, lessening the amount of time and the degree to which the wound is susceptible to cross-contamination and infection. Adhesive gauze or nonadherent, self-adherent, or adherent tapes and wraps can be applied as secondary dressings to secure primary occlusive dressings during athletic activities.

SCENARIO 7

A marathon runner is receiving treatment for patellofemoral pain in the outpatient orthopedic clinic. The patient presents for the biweekly appointment and reports falling on a roadway during a cycling ride since the last visit. After falling, the patient scrubbed the wound with sterile gauze and soap, and no dressing was applied. An assessment reveals an anterior knee abrasion of unknown depth and the development of black, desiccated eschar firmly attached to the wound bed. No clinical signs of infection are present. Based on the information, what actions are appropriate in this situation?

Recommendations

Using the findings (eg, medical history) from the initial knee assessment, evaluate the present abrasion injury. The formation of eschar will restrict the assessment of the wound bed. The immediate goal is the debridement of the eschar to allow for the evaluation of the wound bed, diagnosis of the injury, and creation of a management plan based on the findings. Among the debridement techniques, wet to moist is recommended for eschar removal. The normal saline or potable tap water will donate moisture to the eschar, softening and loosening the material from the wound bed. The eschar will adhere to the woven, sterile gauze and be lifted from the wound bed with dressing removal. Multiple applications of the gauze may be required based on the thickness of the eschar. Maintain the moisture level of the gauze and monitor the periwound tissue for maceration. After removal of the eschar, irrigation with normal saline or potable tap water and autolytic debridement with occlusive dressings can be used to remove the remaining devitalized tissue and waste to promote an optimal healing environment.

Things to Consider

Multiple debridement techniques could be considered in this situation. The choice of a technique is based on patient, wound, and clinician factors and applicable state laws. Eschar and debris adhered to the wound bed can delay healing and increase the risk of infection. Removal will decrease the bacterial bioburden of the wound and prepare a viable wound bed for dressing application. The initial use of autolytic debridement is contraindicated before the removal of the eschar and a thorough assessment, diagnosis, and cleansing of the wound bed. Based on the eschar attachment to the wound bed, the use of conservative sharp, scrubbing, and wet-to-dry techniques could result in trauma to viable tissues and produce pain. The pressure ranges of irrigation are inadequate to penetrate, moisten, and soften the desiccated eschar. Hydrotherapy can moisten and soften the eschar but is not indicated for use with acute skin trauma. Chemical debridement is contraindicated for eschar removal because of possible cytotoxicity to viable tissues. After debridement of the eschar with the wet-to-moist technique, irrigation and autolytic techniques can remove the remaining devitalized tissue and waste to promote a moist, clean, and warm healing environment.

SCENARIO 8

The school administration and athletic training staff are planning for the fall sports parent and guardian meeting scheduled for the summer. The group discusses the development of additional educational resources to promote the health and safety of student athletes. Based on the frequency of acute skin trauma and the best practice interventions used in the management plans, the athletic training staff has experienced multiple episodes of delayed and unreported skin trauma, unnecessary dressing changes, and lack of adherence to daily monitoring, resulting in adverse outcomes. The administration and athletic training staff agree that creating and disseminating a wound care infographic can provide education and improve adherence to management plans among student athletes, parents, and guardians to support healing outcomes. Based on this information, what actions are appropriate in this situation?

Recommendations

The athletic training staff can access published acute skin trauma position and consensus statements and guidelines from health care professions, organizations, and facilities to develop the infographic. The infographic can communicate the purposes, goals, and recommendations for postinjury care in an easy-to-understand format. The infographic could include guidance on reporting, follow-up, and monitoring of skin trauma; cleansing, debridement, and dressing interventions; and when to seek a referral. An example infographic is found in Appendix B.

Things to Consider

Although multiple designs can be considered for the infographic, the contents must be based on the current resources, policies, and procedures and cleansing, debridement, and dressing interventions in the athletic training facility. For example, the recommendations should include only those dressings purchased and used in the management plans. Sufficient personnel must be available to monitor and reassess student athletes daily or on a regular schedule. The use of occlusive dressings in management plans may require additional recommendations for education on their duration of wear and changes in the wound and dressing that occur with the creation of a moist environment. The infographic can also reinforce the importance of adherence to the management plan. Several targeted populations should receive the infographic including school administrators, coaches, teachers, student athletes, parents, and guardians. Printed copies can be distributed at parent and guardian meetings and posted in the athletic training facility, locker rooms, and other high-traffic areas. Electronic infographic communication through email, website, and social media postings is also recommended.

SCENARIO 9

During the renovation of restrooms at a local restaurant, a plumber is refitting the main waterlines with copper tubing. The tubing cutter fails, and the cutting wheel strikes the right thumb. The plumber returns to work immediately postinjury with the thumb covered with an adhesive strip and tape. The patient presents the next day for an evaluation. Past medical history reveals the patient is a smoker and is currently taking nonsteroidal anti-inflammatory medication for a lower back injury sustained 2 weeks ago. Otherwise, the medical history is normal. An assessment of the right thumb demonstrates a partial-thickness laceration with contamination of unknown, small debris. There is mild sanguineous drainage from the laceration and moderate erythema in the periwound tissue. The wound edges are approximated. The laceration is irrigated with normal saline, and the periwound tissue is scrubbed with sterile gauze and a topical antiseptic. A hydrocolloid primary dressing and self-adherent wrap secondary dressing are applied. Patient education is provided on healthy lifestyles and temporary modifications to work activities to protect the wound and promote healing. Reassessments over the next weeks include dressing changes because the outer foam layer of the hydrocolloid begins to break down from repeated exposure to moisture during work activities. The self-adherent wrap secondary dressing is also changed to lessen the risk of periwound maceration. Inspection of the wound bed and periwound tissue reveals dehiscence of the wound edges, persistent erythema, and a lack of progression in healing. Based on this information, what actions are appropriate in this situation?

Recommendations

A thorough, holistic reassessment of the patient, wound bed, periwound tissue, and dressing and a review of past findings should be conducted immediately. Factors associated with an increased risk of infection and adverse reactions identified in the patient medical history and history of the present injury and findings from assessments of the wound bed, periwound tissue, and dressing are critical in guiding treatment. The patient's medical and current injury history revealed several risk factors for infection, and reassessments demonstrated findings inconsistent with expected healing outcomes. Apply sterile gauze over the wound and promptly refer the patient for further assessment of infection.

Things to Consider

All acute skin trauma is initially considered contaminated. Comprehensive assessment and early recognition of the clinical features of infection and adverse reactions will direct appropriate treatment and referral. The wound etiology and patient medical history demonstrated several risk factors associated with infection and adverse reactions. The wound was sustained in a contaminated environment, and appropriate assessment and cleansing and debridement interventions were delayed until the following day. The initial assessment found the wound contaminated with unknown debris. The injury environment, delay in treatment, and foreign material contamination increased the risk of infection. The patient reported a history of smoking and the current use of nonsteroidal anti-inflammatory medication. These lifestyle factors may contribute to a delay in normal healing. The delay in healing increases the time the wound is vulnerable to further contamination and infection. The initial use of nonocclusive adhesive strips and tape is also associated with an increased risk of infection, which is further increased with the immediate return to work in the contaminated environment. Repeated exposure to moisture and saturation of the hydrocolloid and self-adherent wrap can cause maceration and delayed healing. Patient, wound, and intervention factors can contribute to the development of infection and adverse outcomes. The initial presence of multiple risk factors and assessment findings inconsistent with normal healing should heighten awareness for early detection and consideration for the timely referral.

SCENARIO 10

A patient returns from vacation and reports falling at a skateboard park. The patient was seen at an urgent care center and diagnosed with a full-thickness lateral hip abrasion. The wound was cleansed, debrided, and dressed with primary nonadherent pads and secondary adherent tape. An assessment is performed. Inspection of the dressing reveals strike-through and adherence to the wound bed. Leakage has occurred with desiccated exudate on the dressing edges and adherent tape. There is mild erythema and swelling in the periwound tissue, and the patient reports mild pain in the periwound tissue with palpation. The adhered dressing obstructs the assessment of the wound bed. Active hip range of motion is limited by pain over the wound area. The patient's medical history is unremarkable, and clinical features of infection are absent. Based on the information, what actions are appropriate in this situation?

Recommendations

Removal of the nonadherent pads and adherent tape is necessary to assess the wound bed and develop a management plan. The dressing and tape require rehydration before removal attempts to prevent trauma to the wound bed and periwound tissue. Irrigation with normal saline or potable tap water is recommended to rehydrate the dressing and tape. Irrigate until saturated. Keep the dressing and tape soaked and irrigate as needed while the dressing and tape remain in place for a period. The moisture will soften and liquefy the exudate and loosen the nonadherent pads from the wound bed and periwound tissue. Carefully remove the skin from the tape rather than ripping the tape away from the skin. Once the dressing loosens, gently lift the pads from the tissues. Irrigation can be used during removal to help break any remaining adherence. With dressing removal, assess the wound bed to determine the type and color of the tissue, the depth of tissue damage, and contamination. Evaluate the condition of the periwound tissue. Based on the findings, cleanse, debride, and dress the wound within the management plan.

Things to Consider

The initial evaluation revealed several findings to guide dressing selection and the management plan. Full-thickness abrasions involve trauma through the epidermis, dermis, and into subcutaneous tissues and produce moderate to heavy amounts of exudate. The assessment demonstrated the production of heavy exudate and saturation of the dressing that resulted in strike-through and subsequent leakage. Dressings should promote healing, prevent adverse reactions, lessen pain, manage exudate, and protect the wound. Although several nonocclusive and occlusive dressings are indicated for full-thickness wounds, their use should follow application and wear guidelines. Nonocclusive dressings require daily changes to lessen the risk of adverse reactions present in the scenario. Failure of the nonadherent pads to manage the exudate and possible delayed dressing changes increased the risk of cross-contamination and infection and allowed desiccation and adherence of the dressing to the wound bed, which can delay healing. If occlusive dressings are available, consider alginates or foams designed to manage copious amounts of exudate, create a moist environment, promote healing, lessen adverse events, and protect the wound. Regardless of the dressing type chosen, daily monitoring and reassessment and patient education can reduce the risk of dressing compromise (eg, strike-through, saturation, and leakage) and wound desiccation and guide modifications to interventions in the management plan.

SCENARIO 11

A lacrosse attacker is tripped while taking a shot; falls on the artificial turf field; and sustains a partial-thickness lateral, distal upper arm and elbow abrasion. After a sideline assessment and cleansing and dressing interventions, the patient returns to the game. After the game, a thorough assessment is completed and is unremarkable. The abrasion is cleansed, debrided, and dressed with a nonocclusive adhesive patch. Topical neomycin is applied to the wound bed under the dressing to lower the risk of infection and promote a moist wound environment. A reassessment and dressing change with the application of neomycin are performed daily. Three days postinjury, the patient presents with pruritis, erythema, edema, and mild pain localized on the periwound tissue covered by the adhesive patch. Based on the symptoms, the timing of the symptoms, and the setting of the injury (eg, artificial turf field), the patient is referred for an assessment of infection. The results of the assessment are negative. Although the patient reported no known allergies, the adhesive of the dressing edges is the suspected cause of the symptoms. The adhesive patch is discontinued, and a nonadherent pad and neomycin are applied. The patient returns the following day with worsening erythema, edema, and pain and eruption of vesicles on the periwound tissue. Based on this information, what actions are appropriate in this situation?

Recommendations

The symptoms, interventions, and negative infection diagnosis likely indicate the patient has developed allergic contact dermatitis. Allergic contact dermatitis is caused by contact with or exposure to an allergen. The allergen should be identified and discontinued in the management plan. In this scenario, neomycin is the likely offending source of the symptoms. Referral and patch testing can confirm neomycin as the causative allergen. Remove the neomycin from the wound bed with normal saline or potable tap water irrigation. Wet-to-moist debridement of the wound bed may also be considered. If necessary, use sterile gauze premoistened with normal saline or potable tap water to gently scrub neomycin from the periwound tissue. Apply topical corticosteroids to the area as directed by a physician and reassess the dressing selection. Nonadhesive, nonocclusive dressings may be initially preferable based on the daily changes required for the application of the topical corticosteroid and monitoring and reassessment of symptoms. With a reduction of symptoms and integrity of the periwound tissue, occlusive dressings are indicated to provide a barrier to the external environment to lessen the risk of contamination and infection. A referral is warranted with persistent, worsening, or developing emergent symptoms.

Things to Consider

The mechanism of injury (eg, artificial turf field), unremarkable medical history (eg, allergies), assessment, and dressing choice supported the use of topical antimicrobials to reduce the risk of infection. However, the repeated application of neomycin resulted in an allergic reaction and disruption of the skin's barrier properties. The clinical features of allergic contact dermatitis, erythema, edema, pain, and vesicles are similar to developing an infection. Additionally, the greatest concern for infection is immediately postinjury, which coincides with the time topical antibiotics are commonly applied. Referral for the assessment of infection should be considered. Comprehensive monitoring and reassessment of the patient and the wound can identify the development of adverse reactions and direct referral for symptoms inconsistent with physical findings. The recommended cleansing and debridement techniques can effectively remove the neomycin without causing trauma to the healing tissues. Other cleansing and debridement techniques, such as hydrotherapy, scrubbing and swabbing, wet-to-dry, and chemical debridement, are contraindicated based on the nonselective removal and cytotoxicity to viable tissues and increase the risk of contamination and infection.

Occlusive dressings are favored over nonocclusive dressings for lowering the rates of infection. However, the condition of the periwound tissue can prevent the use of occlusive dressings initially. Occlusion of the periwound tissue and excessive adhesion of the dressings can result in further irritation and trauma to the area. With the improvement of symptoms and healing of the periwound tissue, occlusive dressings can be considered.

SCENARIO 12

A landscaper loses control of a gas hedge trimmer and sustains a full-thickness palmar laceration to the left third finger between the proximal and distal interphalangeal joints. The patient was taken to an emergency department for assessment and wound closure. After the assessment, which is otherwise unremarkable, the laceration is cleansed, debrided, and closed with nonabsorbable sutures. A sterile gauze secondary dressing is applied. The patient returns on postinjury day 9 for suture removal and is allowed to resume work activities as tolerated. The next day, the patient operates a string trimmer and pinches the left third finger in the handle. The patient presents at the outpatient clinic, and the assessment demonstrates partial dehiscence in the laceration, mild serosanguinous drainage, and no clinical features of infection. The dehisced edges of the laceration can be manually approximated, and the superficial- to partial-thickness wound bed reveals granulation tissue. The laceration undergoes cleansing and debridement. The patient desires to return to work as soon as possible. Based on this information, what actions are appropriate in this situation?

Recommendations

Although the initial assessment in the emergency department did not reveal any comorbidities that may affect wound healing (eg, medications, smoking, or diabetes), consider referral of the patient to rule out any factors that may contribute to dehiscence. Pressure on the laceration from the string trimmer handle and early removal of the sutures in an area of high skin tension likely led to the dehiscence. Based on the partial dehiscence and wound depth, sutures are not indicated for closure. Wound closure strips or dermal adhesives can be used to approximate the wound edges. Apply a secondary dressing such as sterile gauze or nonadherent pads and adhesive gauze or nonadherent, self-adherent, or adherent tape or wrap to protect the wound and the closure method from pressure and friction during work activities. A felt or foam donut pad and nonsterile hydrogel can also lessen friction and pressure forces over the laceration. Replace the secondary dressings when wet and remove them overnight to reduce the risk of periwound tissue maceration. Patient guidance and education can improve healing outcomes and should be included in the management plan. Communicate and develop temporary modifications in work activities with the patient to lessen shear and tensile forces and loads on the wound and dressing to maintain wound closure and promote complete healing.

Things to Consider

Wound dehiscence can increase the risk of infection and delay healing, and prompt assessment and consideration of referral are warranted. The palmar finger laceration was between the proximal and distal interphalangeal joints and was subjected to high skin tension with finger flexion and extension during work activities. In this location of high tension and stress, the sutures should remain in place and be removed after 10 to 14 days to support tissue approximation and allow further healing. The application of wound closure strips following the day 9 suture removal could also assist in maintaining tissue approximation. Patient education in this situation should focus on wound closure goals and work activity modifications. Clinician communication and education on the management plan will promote patient adherence to achieve healing outcomes.

SCENARIO 13

The annual athletic training supply and equipment budget for the upcoming fiscal year is near completion. The athletic director approaches and states the supply budget needs to be cut by 20%. A needs assessment and revising the supply list remove many items, including those used in acute wound care. The inventory is adequate to support cleansing and debridement interventions in the management plans. Nonocclusive primary dressings and adhesive gauze and nonadherent, self-adherent, and adherent tapes and wraps used as secondary dressings are sufficient. However, the variety and types of occlusive dressings normally purchased must be reduced. Based on this information, what actions are appropriate in this situation?

Recommendations

Dressings are constructed with a variety of materials and designed for specific purposes. Dressing selection is determined by characteristics of the wound and patient and the availability of dressings. Most cases of acute skin trauma sustained among athletes are superficial- to partial-thickness wounds that require secondary closure with primary dressings. Patient characteristics in this setting commonly include a low incidence of comorbidities, healthy lifestyles, and outdoor and indoor sports participation. Based on these selection factors and the budget restriction, film and hydrocolloid dressings are appropriate choices. Films are indicated as primary dressings for superficial- to partial-thickness wounds with low amounts of exudate. Film dressings are flexible and possess the ability to adhere to most body contours. Hydrocolloids are indicated as primary dressings with partial- to full-thickness wounds with minimal to moderate exudate levels. These conformable dressings are thicker in construction and can be cut into various sizes and shapes. Adhesive gauze and nonadherent, self-adherent, and adherent tapes and wraps can be used as secondary dressings to maintain adherence of the films and hydrocolloids to the periwound tissue during practices and competitions.

Things to Consider

No one nonocclusive or occlusive dressing is appropriate for every wound, and few dressings are suited for a single wound to promote an optimal environment throughout the healing process. Although this statement implies the purchase and availability of a wide selection of dressings for facilities, the budget cut limited the selection of occlusive dressings. In this spending reduction situation, dressings were selected and purchased based on the wound and patient characteristics. Past injury data can identify the frequency and types of acute skin trauma sustained and dressing types used in management plans. Film and hydrocolloid dressings are appropriate for use with athletes because their construction and integrity are sufficient to withstand sports demands and changing environmental conditions. Nonocclusive dressings can be considered for management plans despite the slower rates of healing and the higher risk of infection compared to occlusive dressings. Occlusive dressings may also be cost-effective when compared to nonocclusive dressings in the management of noninfected wounds. For example, a soccer athlete sustains a partial-thickness lateral forearm abrasion during the season. During a typical week, team practices are held Monday, Tuesday, Wednesday, and Friday, with Thursday and Saturday matches. Sunday is an off day. A film or nonadherent pad can be applied as the primary dressing. Secondary dressings for the film include adhesive gauze applied on the borders of the dressing and nonadherent wrap covering the film for practices and matches. Sterile gauze pads and nonadherent wrap serve as secondary dressings with the nonadherent pad to absorb exudate and secure the dressing over the wound. An additional nonadherent wrap is applied with the nonadherent pad for practices and matches. In the absence of clinical features of infection or adverse reactions, the film can remain in place for 7 days; the nonadherent pad requires changes after morning and postpractice and match showering. Additional changes of the nonadherent pad may be necessary if the dressing becomes saturated with exudate. The approximate costs of the dressings over 7 days are as follows.

Primary Dressing	Primary Dressing
Film $2.18 each $2.18 over 7 days	Nonadherent pad $.20 each, 2/day, $.40 $2.80 over 7 days
Secondary Dressing	**Secondary Dressing**
Adhesive gauze $.60 per 12 inches (cut strips widthwise) $.60 over 7 days	Sterile gauze pads $.08 each (3 pads per dressing change, 2/day), $.48 $3.36 over 7 days
Nonadherent wrap $1.57 roll, 3/rolls (< 1/2 roll for practice/match) $4.71 over 7 days	Nonadherent wrap $1.57 roll, 9/rolls (< 1/2 roll for home, < 1/2 roll practice/match) $14.13 over 7 days
Total 7 days	**Total 7 days**
$7.49	$20.29

Along with the reduced costs of the actual primary and secondary dressings, occlusive dressings may lower the costs of applying the dressings based on fewer changes, lower the overall clinician time required to treat the wound based on faster rates of healing, and lower the risk of infection compared with nonocclusive dressings.

SCENARIO 14

An elementary schoolteacher presents to the clinic with an open blister over the thenar eminence. The patient reports a nonsignificant medical history; an active lifestyle participating in cycling, strength training, and motocross; no previous injury to the hand; and no complications with past skin trauma interventions and healing. The patient reports the injury was sustained yesterday while riding motocross at the track from repeated shear forces between loose-fitting gloves and gripping of the handlebars. The pain is moderate and localized to the wound bed. No other symptoms are reported. The patient states the wound was initially cleansed with tap water and covered with an adhesive patch. Since the injury, no changes in the level of pain or the amount of drainage have been noted. An inspection reveals a 2.50 cm × 2.50 cm open blister with exposed granulation tissue of partial-thickness depth over the thenar eminence. Small quantities of debris and denuded tissue are present in the wound bed with moderate exudate and serous drainage. Mild erythema is present in the periwound tissue. A necrotic skin flap is loosely attached to 50% of the wound perimeter. Palpation of soft tissues and the surrounding structures is unremarkable. The active range of motion and functional ability of the thumb are limited secondary to pain. Neurologic and vascular assessments and a review of systems are nonsignificant. The clinical diagnosis is a partial-thickness thenar eminence open blister. Based on this information, what actions are appropriate in this situation?

Recommendations

The development of a management plan is warranted. The plan should contain cleansing, debridement, and dressing interventions; the frequency of reassessments; patient education; the prognosis of healing and return to activity; and goals. The initial interventions and associated patient education in a sample plan are presented.

Cleansing

Goal: The removal of all visible debris and nonadherent denuded tissue from the wound bed and debris from the periwound tissue and the reduction of bacterial bioburden of the periwound tissue with a topical antiseptic

Technique: Irrigate the wound bed and periwound tissue with normal saline or potable tap water. Continue irrigation to remove all visible debris. Scrubbing of the periwound tissue with sterile gauze or foam sponge soaked with normal saline, potable tap water, or topical antiseptic can be performed. Avoid contact of the gauze or sponge with the wound bed.

Patient Education: Irrigation will remove loose debris and microorganisms from the wound bed without damaging the healing tissues. After the initial cleansing, cleanse the wound bed only if it becomes visibly contaminated or demonstrates clinical features of infection or adverse reactions. Avoid repeated cleansing of the wound bed.

Debridement

Goal: The removal of the loosely attached necrotic tissue on the wound perimeter

Technique: With sterile instruments, remove the necrotic flap along the border between the nonviable and viable tissue with the conservative sharp technique. Verify state laws and practice acts before performing. Irrigate the wound bed with normal saline or potable tap water after debridement of the necrotic flap.

Patient Education: Fully explain the conservative sharp procedure and the use of sharp instruments and obtain patient consent before performing. Removing necrotic tissue reduces the bacterial bioburden, lessens the risk of infection, and prepares the wound for dressing application.

Dressing

Goal: Support and promote healing, prevent contamination and infection, and protect the wound

Technique: Nonocclusive and occlusive dressings can be considered. Occlusive dressings are recommended. A hydrocolloid or hydrogel primary dressing is indicated to manage the moderate exudate. Cut the hydrocolloid to extend 1 to 2 cm beyond the wound bed if the palmar hand size allows. Cut the hydrogel to the size of the wound. Adhesive gauze can be applied over the hydrocolloid as a secondary dressing. A secondary film dressing can adhere the hydrogel to the periwound tissue. Adhesive gauze can be applied on the borders of the film to enhance adherence. Nonadherent, self-adherent, or adherent tapes and wraps can be used as additional secondary dressings with the hydrocolloid and hydrogel.

Patient Education: The hydrocolloid dressing will interact with the wound exudate to form a gel, creating a moist environment, insulating the wound, and protecting the healing tissues. It is normal for the dressing to swell or expand over the wound as the moist environment develops. The hydrogel dressing will absorb exudate and promote a moist wound environment. A brownish fluid may be visible over the wound as the moist environment is created. The fluid is expected with the hydrogel dressing. The hydrocolloid dressing can remain over the wound bed for 5 to 7 days and the hydrogel for 1 to 7 days. Unnecessary dressing changes can delay healing. The secondary dressings will be monitored and changed when needed during reassessments. Bathing and showering are allowed with the dressings in place. However, avoid soaking the dressings. Occlusive dressings and a moist wound environment produce faster rates of healing and lower rates of infection compared to nonocclusive dressings. The hydrocolloid and hydrogel dressings and moist environment will also use the body's mechanisms to promote autolytic debridement to remove necrotic tissue and waste from the wound bed and support healing.

After cleansing, debridement, and dressing interventions, provide patient education on the management plan's goals, reassessments, expected healing time and return to activity, and self-monitoring. The overall goal of the management plan is to create an optimal (eg, clean, moist, and warm) wound environment to achieve complete healing in the shortest amount of time. Healing of the partial-thickness open blister should occur within weeks with a return to work activities as tolerated. A return to cycling, strength training, and motocross can be considered with a low risk of reinjury, full functional ability, and met objectives of the interventions. Reassessments of your condition and wound, dressing, and healing should occur daily or regularly based on your availability. Follow the guidelines in the management plan and self-monitor the wound area for signs and symptoms of infection and adverse reactions. Immediately contact the clinic if pain, drainage, warmth, redness, or swelling worsen or rash, fever, itching, or leakage from the dressing develop. Review the management plan guidelines with the patient and ask if they have any concerns or questions.

Things to Consider

The management plan's initial interventions, goals, and patient education were based on the assessment findings and clinical diagnosis. The management plan will evolve during the progression of healing. Modifications to the plan are often required to correspond to the effects of cleansing, debridement, and dressing interventions on healing, patient functional goals, and the development of adverse reactions. Monitoring and reassessing the patient, wound bed, periwound tissue, and dressing(s) on a daily or regular schedule will guide dressing changes and revisions to the plan to achieve patient and healing outcomes. Generally, additional wound bed cleansing during the progression of normal healing is unnecessary. Irrigation may be considered to rehydrate the wound, lessen trauma when removing a dressing adhered to the wound, or visually inspect the wound. Continued cleansing of the wound is required with clinical features of infection. A viable wound bed can be created with the initial debridement of the necrotic tissue with the conservative sharp technique. Occlusive dressings and a moist wound environment support autolytic debridement of any remaining necrotic tissue, and further debridement is not warranted. Selecting an occlusive dressing for the partial-thickness blister will require dressing transitions in the management plan. Transitions are based on patient, wound, and dressing factors and changes in the wound bed produced by the progression of healing.

SUMMARY

Managing acute skin trauma requires the clinician to simultaneously consider and evaluate numerous factors and components, beginning with the initial assessment through complete healing. The selection of cleansing, debridement, and dressing interventions and the development of a management plan that will promote healing and lessen adverse reactions are based on patient, wound, and clinician factors and the types and availability of supplies. Daily monitoring and reassessment of the patient, wound, periwound tissue, and dressing and patient education are critical components in the management plan to achieve healing outcomes. Determining the specific interventions to select and perform within the management plan can be challenging. These decisions should be approached in a holistic manner and supported by the best available research evidence and literature, the clinician's experience, and the patient's goals and needs. The appropriate management of acute skin trauma is essential in the practice of athletic training. Simulated learning strategies such as scenarios provide the opportunity for clinicians to develop clinical decision-making skills among various populations and settings in a controlled environment.

GLOSSARY

A

Anaphylaxis: immediate, severe reaction from sensitization following prior contact to an allergen with local or systemic reaction and symptoms; can be fatal.

Antiseptics: agents used to eradicate or reduce the number of microorganisms in a wound; also known as antimicrobials.

B

Bullae: large vesicles created by the separation of the epidermis from the subepidermal structure and typically filled with fluid.

C

Channels: the progression of exudate from the wound bed to the perimeter of a film dressing.

Cleaning: to remove dirt and gross debris from a person, surface, or object.

Clean technique: infection control procedure to lessen the overall number of microorganisms and lower rates of transmission by using sterile instruments and clean supplies and equipment.

Contaminated: presence or introduction of infectious agent onto a normally clean person, surface, or object.

D

Decontaminated: to remove or destroy microorganisms from a person, surface, or object.

Dehiscence: opening of wound margins or edges.

Denuded: removal of skin or tissue through trauma.

Desiccated: dry, absence of moisture.

Devitalized: deprived of life or vitality.

Disinfection: to destroy or inactivate microorganisms on inanimate objects.

E

Ecchymosis: superficial black and blue discoloration of the skin from hemorrhage.

Eczematous: skin marked by redness, itching, and weeping lesions that may become thickened and crusted.

Edematous: related to excessive swelling and fluid accumulation in tissues.

Erythema: reddening of the skin caused by trauma or inflammation.

Erythematous: skin marked by erythema.

Eschar: black or brown devitalized tissue; a scab.

Exothermic: reaction that releases heat.

Exotoxins: toxins or poisonous substances produced and secreted by bacteria.

Exudate: fluid, cells, protein, and solids released from blood vessels into tissues following trauma.

F

Fluctuance: wavelike sensation felt on palpation of the skin produced by the presence of fluid (eg, pus).

G

Granulation tissue: temporary connective tissue consisting of fibroblasts, capillaries, and cells in wounds healing by secondary intention.

I

Immunocompromised: having a weakened immune system caused by disease or drugs.

Inanimate: absence of life, lifeless.

Induration: a firmness or hardening of tissue.

Infectious: ability to be transmitted and produce infection.

L

Lymphadenopathy: disease process of the lymph nodes usually causing enlargement.

Lymphangitis: inflammation of the lymphatic vessels.

M

Maceration: softening of the skin by wetting; skin is white in appearance.

Mitotic activity: reproduction of cells essential to healing.

Mucocutaneous junctions: boundary where mucosa transitions to skin (eg, lips and eye).

Mucosal surfaces: surfaces and cavities lined with epithelial cells (eg, mouth and nose).

N

Necrotic: dead or dying.

Nonpurulent: absence of pus.

No-touch technique: infection control procedure in which no portion of a dressing that contacts the wound bed is touched during application.

P

Periwound tissue: area of skin that is 4 cm beyond the wound edges.

Potable tap water: water that is considered safe to drink.

Primary closure: wound healing through primary intention when the wound edges can be approximated.

Primary dressing: wound dressing placed directly on the wound bed.

Pruritic: associated with itching.

Pruritus: itching; sensation can be intense or severe.

Purulent: forming or composed of pus.

S

Sanguineous: fluid containing blood.

Secondary closure: wound healing through secondary intention with a dressing covering the wound and formation of granulation tissue.

Secondary dressing: wound dressing used with a primary dressing to provide occlusion, absorption, adherence, and protection for the wound bed.

Serosanguinous: fluid relating to blood and serum.

Serous: thin, watery fluid resembling serum.

Slough: moist, fibrous devitalized tissue.

Slough off: to separate or fall off.

Splash back: solution striking the wound bed and returning toward the patient and clinician during irrigation.

Standard precautions: infection control guidelines that assume all patients are potentially infected or colonized with microorganisms that can be transmitted.

Stellate: shape of a star.

Sterile technique: infection control procedure to lessen exposure to microorganisms by using sterile instruments, supplies, and equipment.

Sterilization: to destroy all microorganisms on a surface or object.

Strike-through: leakage of exudate from the wound bed through the dressing; visible on the outer dressing layer.

Surgical debridement: removal of viable or nonviable tissue, foreign material, and debris from the wound bed in a sterile environment.

T

Tissue approximation: bring or draw tissues together.

Tunnel: a channel that extends from any part of the wound and continues into deeper tissue.

U

Universal precautions: infection control guidelines that assume all blood and body fluid are infectious.

Urticaria: raised rash on the skin; hives.

Urticarial: an allergic reaction producing hives or wheals on the skin.

V

Vesicles: small fluid-filled sacs on the skin, blisterlike.

Viable: living, ability to survive and develop.

A

WOUND CLOSURE

The management of traumatic lacerations and incisions and postoperative incisions that require tissue approximation is accomplished through several techniques. Wounds in areas of minimal static and dynamic skin tension can be managed with wound closure strips or dermal adhesives. Lacerations and incisions with jagged edges, edges that cannot be approximated, or exposed subcutaneous tissue or located over a joint, in areas with high skin tension, or excessive moisture production require more advanced closure methods.[1,2] Sutures and staples are used with these wounds to provide hemostasis, eliminate dead space, prevent infection, approximate tissues, restore function, and achieve optimal healing and cosmetic outcomes.[2,3] These techniques require knowledge of anatomy, wound healing, and overall management plan and the necessary skill and confidence in performing the techniques obtained through professional training.

State laws and practice acts regulate the use of sutures and staples for wound closure. Rules and regulations differ among states regarding what techniques and procedures are allowed. Clinicians should carefully review applicable state laws and practice acts before performing wound closure with sutures and staples. In states that prohibit or do not address these techniques, clinicians must refer the patient to an appropriately credentialed provider for treatment. This discussion includes common suture and staple techniques for the management of lacerations and incisions. The techniques are presented to evolve with changes in educational standards in professions and state practice acts and guide current clinical practice in various settings.[4]

Wound closure with sutures and staples is performed with the sterile technique including handwashing; creating and maintaining a sterile field; and the use of sterile personal protective equipment, instruments, and supplies. Cleaning and disinfecting surfaces, equipment, and laundry and disposal of medical waste must adhere to facility policies and guidelines. See Chapter 2 for a discussion on infection control guidelines.

SUTURES

The clinical decision to suture follows a thorough assessment of the patient and cleansing and possible wound debridement. The patient assessment should include a health history of tetanus vaccination and allergies to closure materials. Irrigation, sharp, and **surgical debridement** techniques for the removal of embedded foreign debris or viable or nonviable tissue require referral of the patient to a physician. Clinicians must consider the suture material, size, and needle and suture technique to achieve healing and cosmetic outcomes.[3]

Sutures are classified based on the suture material (absorbable vs nonabsorbable), structure (monofilament vs multifilament), and origin (synthetic vs natural) (Table A-1). Absorbable sutures are naturally digested by the body over a general period of 4 to 8 weeks and do not require removal. Some types can take up to 6 months to dissolve. Absorbable sutures are often used for deep, multilayer lacerations[2] to decrease dead space and tension on the wound edges for tissue approximation. Absorbable sutures can also be used in low-tension wounds and when it may be difficult to remove sutures.[5] Nonabsorbable sutures require eventual removal after tissue closure, provide greater tensile strength, and cause less tissue reactivity. A monofilament suture is a simple thread of suture material that easily passes through tissues, causing less trauma. These sutures possess higher memory, making them difficult to handle and tie. Multifilament sutures are pliable braided or twisted fibers, possess high tensile strength, and have less memory for easier handling during techniques. Multifilament sutures produce more friction passing through tissues, increasing the risk of inflammation and infection at the site. Synthetic sutures are manufactured from polyamide, hydrocarbon, or propylene polymers and cause less of an inflammatory reaction than natural sutures. Natural sutures are manufactured from animal tissues and are associated with a greater risk of inflammation at the suture site. Natural sutures possess a variable distribution of tensile strength compared with synthetic sutures.

Suture sizes are based on the diameter of the material. Sizes from 0 to 7 represent increasingly thicker material, with 7 possessing the largest diameter. Suture sizes from 2-0 to 11-0 indicate smaller diameter material, with 11-0 being the thinnest in diameter. Sizes typically used for lacerations range from 3-0 to 6-0. Generally, sutures with a larger diameter have greater tensile strength, produce a larger hole, and cause greater tissue damage. Size selection of the suture material is based on wound location and tissue condition, skin thickness and tension, the potential for infection and adverse reactions, and patient health status. The overall goal is to select the smallest suture size that will approximate the wound edges and close the wound to produce acceptable healing and cosmetic

Table A-1. Suture Types

Absorbable	Polyglactin 910 Polydioxanone Poliglecaprone 25 Surgical gut (plain, chromic, fast absorbing)
Nonabsorbable	Nylon Polypropylene Polyester Stainless steel Silk
Monofilament	Polypropylene Nylon Polyester Poliglecaprone 25 Polydioxanone
Multifilament	Polyglactin 910 Silk (braided) Polyester (braided)
Synthetic	Polyglactin 910 Poliglecaprone 25 Polydioxanone Nylon Polypropylene
Natural	Surgical gut Silk

Table A-2. Suture Size Guidelines

Body region	Suture Size
Scalp	3-0 to 5-0
Face/lips	5-0 to 6-0
Trunk	4-0 to 5-0
Extremities	4-0 to 5-0
Hands	4-0 to 5-0
Feet	3-0 to 4-0

Table A-3. Common Suture Techniques[2,7,9]

Simple interrupted	• Most commonly used technique
	• Versatile and easy
	• More time-consuming than other techniques
	• Used for linear or irregular traumatic and postoperative wounds
	• Effective for deep wounds
	• Consists of individual strands of material
	• Approximation remains with breakage of a single strand
	• Produces eversion of wound edges
Horizontal mattress	• Used for gaping and high-tension wounds
	• Effective for calloused areas of skin (soles of feet, palms)
	• Tension is spread among all wound edges
	• Compresses wound edges for hemostasis
	• Produces eversion of wound edges
	• Reduces risk of necrosis
Vertical mattress	• Produces better eversion of wound edges than other techniques
	• Used for thick or thin skin
	• Provides secure grasp of tissue and good approximation
	• Used for wounds under tension
	• Increases risk of hatch mark scars
Running continuous	• Used for long, linear, low-tension wounds
	• Allows for more rapid closure than other techniques
	• Produces even distribution of tension along wound
	• Failure in any part of suture will comprise the entire suture

outcomes. See Table A-2 for suture size guidelines based on body region. However, smaller diameter sutures may need to be placed closer together to close the wound.

Suture needles insert the suture material through the tissue. Suture needles have 3 parts: the eye, body, and point.[6] The suture material attaches to the eye; most needles are swaged, with the suture manufactured into the eye.[7] The body of a suture needle can be straight or curved. The circle of the curved body is available in different lengths. A curved needle with a 3/8 circle is most commonly used for skin closure.[6,8] The needle point is commonly a cutting or tapered tip. Cutting needles have 3 cutting edges and are available in standard or reverse cutting designs.[8] These needles penetrate tough tissues such as skin.[8] Tapered needles are round and taper to a point. Tapered needles separate tissues to insert the suture and are used with tissues that do not resist needle penetration, including subcutaneous fat and fascia.[7]

The suture technique is used to mechanically approximate the tissue edges and close the wound in various patterns. Clinicians can determine the most effective technique for closure based on the wound type, length, and location; amount of skin tension; and clinician skill, experience, and comfort with the technique. Table A-3 lists common suture techniques available to clinicians. See Table A-4 for the single interrupted suture technique, perhaps the most commonly used for closure. The sequence of suture placement varies among clinicians. Initial suture placement can begin over the middle section of the wound and then alternate on each side toward the wound ends. Initial suture placement can also begin approximately one-third from the wound edge on one side and then

Table A-4. Simple Interrupted Suture on a Wound Model

- The needle holder is typically held with the dominant hand. Forceps are held in the nondominant hand.
- Load the needle holder by grasping the suture needle one-third from the needle eye with the tip of the needle holder (Figure A-1A).

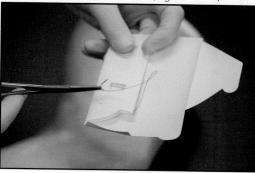

Figure A-1A

- Gently evert (lift) the wound edge with forceps, place the needle perpendicular (90 degrees) to the skin, and pierce the skin with the needle (Figure A-1B).

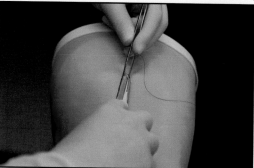

Figure A-1B

- Supinate the wrist and pass the needle through the skin (Figure A-1C). The needle should travel perpendicular to the subcutaneous tissues.

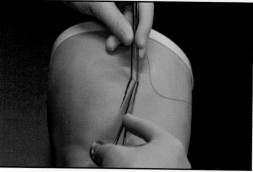

Figure A-1C

continued

Table A-4. Simple Interrupted Suture on a Wound Model (continued)

- Gently evert the skin on the opposing wound edge with forceps and continue to supinate the wrist to push the needle through the skin (Figure A-1D). Release the skin and grasp the suture needle with forceps.

Figure A-1D

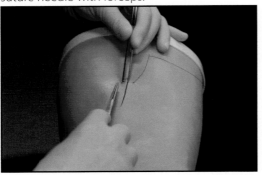

- Pull the suture through both wound edges and leave 2 to 3 cm of the suture material exposed (Figure A-1E). The stitch should be as wide as it is deep.

Figure A-1E

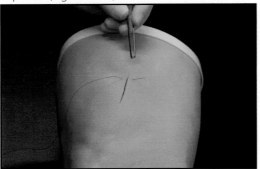

- Hold the needle holder in the dominant hand and the long end of the suture between the nondominant thumb and second finger (Figure A-1F).

Figure A-1F

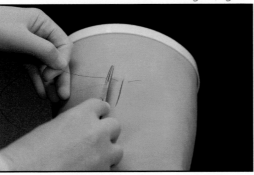

continued

Table A-4. Simple Interrupted Suture on a Wound Model (continued)

- Loop the long end of the suture around the tip of the needle holder twice in a clockwise direction (Figure A-1G).

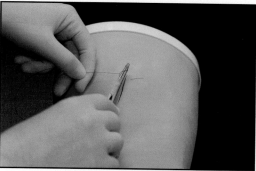

Figure A-1G

- Grasp the exposed, short end of the suture with the needle holder (Figure A-1H).

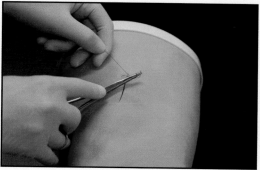

Figure A-1H

- Pull the short end of the suture through the loops on the needle holder by moving the hands in opposite directions with enough tension to close the wound and secure the throw (Figure A-1I).

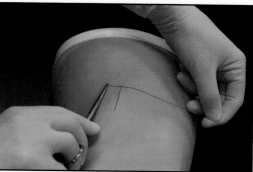

Figure A-1I

continued

Table A-4. Simple Interrupted Suture on a Wound Model (continued)

- Release the suture from the needle holder and continue to hold the long end of the suture with the nondominant thumb and finger.
- Loop the long end of the suture around the needle holder once in a counterclockwise motion (Figure A-1J).

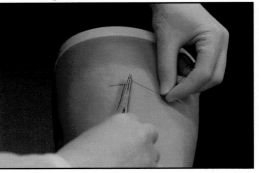

Figure A-1J

- Grasp the short end of the suture with the needle holder and then pull the hands in opposite directions to secure the second throw (Figure A-1K).

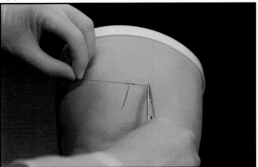

Figure A-1K

- Continue with 2 to 3 additional individual loop throws in the clockwise/counterclockwise pattern.
- Following the throws, cut the suture with scissors, leaving 3 to 4 mm tails (Figure A-1L).

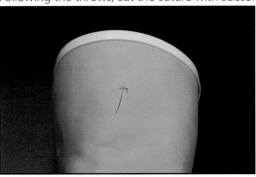

Figure A-1L

- Continue with the procedure until wound closure is complete.
- At completion of the technique, use the needle holder to pull each knot to one side of the wound, away from the laceration or incision.

Table A-5. Suture Removal Time

Body Region	Days
Scalp	6-8
Face/lips	3-5
Trunk	7-10[a]
Extremities	7-10[a]
Hands	7-10[a]
Feet	7-14[a]

[a]Ten to 14 days with lacerations and incisions over joints or in areas of high skin tension.

continue with placement one-third from the opposite edge. Sutures continue in this alternate pattern until wound closure. Sutures are typically spaced 2 to 4 mm apart.

After closure, irrigate the wound with normal saline and pat the area dry with sterile gauze. Clinicians can immobilize wounds over joints to prevent excessive skin tension. Cover the wound with a secondary dressing based on patient needs and activity. Numerous nonocclusive and occlusive dressings can be used with sutured wounds. An evidence-based review demonstrated no findings to support the best nonocclusive or occlusive dressing for postoperative incisions healing by primary intention (tissue approximation using sutures, staples, dermal adhesives, or a combination of these) to lower the rates of infection.[10] Clinicians may select cost-effective nonocclusive designs such as sterile gauze or nonadherent pads to protect the wound and sutures. The sutured wound is often protected from showering and dressing changes for 24 to 48 hours. The authors of an evidence-based review examining early showering (on or before day 2) and delayed showering (after day 3) reported no differences in the rates of infection among postoperative incisions.[11] Clinicians should monitor and reassess the patient and wound daily for intervention outcomes and the development of adverse reactions.

Nonabsorbable sutures are removed based on the healing of the wound and the duration of time in place (Table A-5). A suture removal kit or sterile suture scissors and tweezers or forceps are needed for the technique. The clinician should use the clean technique for the procedure. If applicable, remove the secondary dressing from the wound. Gently scrub the laceration or incision site with sterile gauze premoistened with a topical antiseptic. Irrigation or wet-to-moist debridement with normal saline or potable tap water can be used to soften the dried crust adhered to the sutures or wound site. Pat the wound dry with sterile gauze and remove the sutures (Table A-6). After suture removal, wound closure strips can be applied to support the healing tissues.[3] The use of wound closure strips should be considered with athletes and active patients involved in movements that may produce high skin tension across the wound site.

Table A-6. Suture Removal on a Wound Model

- Using tweezers or forceps, grasp the knot and gently lift the suture (Figure A-2A).

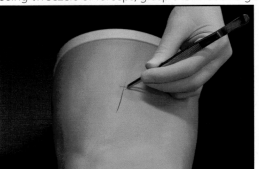

Figure A-2A

- Place the curved tip of the suture scissors under the suture close to the skin (Figure A-2B) and cut (Figure A-2C).

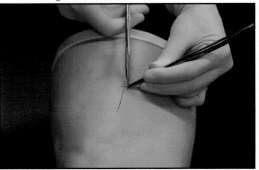

Figure A-2B

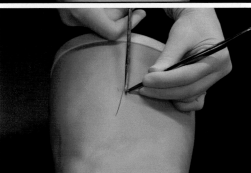

Figure A-2C

continued

Table A-6. Suture Removal on a Wound Model (continued)

- Slowly pull the suture out of the tissues with tweezers or forceps (Figure A-2D).

Figure A-2D

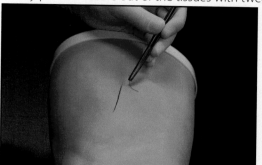

- Place each removed suture on gauze and count the total to ensure removal of all sutures.

STAPLES

Stainless steel staples are an option for wound closure based on the patient's assessment and wound condition following cleansing and debridement. Staples are indicated for the closure of linear lacerations and incisions on the scalp, trunk, and extremities[2] and wounds that are not conducive for suturing.[9] Staples are inappropriate for wounds on the hands, feet, and face because of increased pain with pressure and potential poor cosmetic outcomes. Staples are preloaded and dispensed through a stapler. Staples are available in 2 sizes based on their width, regular and wide. See Table A-7 for the staple technique. Staple placement begins at one end of the wound and progresses toward the other. Staples are generally placed 5 to 10 mm apart over the wound. Care of the patient and wound following closure with staples mimics the guidelines used with sutures.

The removal of staples is performed with a skin staple remover tool. Remove staples in the scalp at 7 days and trunk and extremity staples at 10 days. The clean technique is used for removal. Remove the dressing if in place, gently scrub the wound site with sterile gauze premoistened with a topical antiseptic, then pat dry the area, and remove the staples (Table A-8). Wound closure strips can be applied after the removal of staples if warranted.

SUMMARY

Several options are available to clinicians for the closure of traumatic lacerations and incisions and postoperative incisions. Two methods, sutures and staples, are more advanced closure techniques and may be regulated by state laws and practice acts. Clinicians should review applicable regulations before using sutures and staples for wound closure. The techniques are presented to align with educational standards and to serve as a resource for practicing clinicians involved in wound closure. Wound closure with sutures and staples requires knowledge of anatomy, wound healing, wound management interventions, and training and practice with the techniques.

Table A-7. Staple Technique on a Wound Model

- Approximate and evert the wound edges with forceps or the nondominant thumb and first finger.
- A second clinician can assist with tissue approximation.
- Position the stapler upright (90 degrees) to the skin and over the center of the wound with gentle pressure (Figure A-3A). The depth of staple placement in the skin is determined by the amount of downward pressure applied to the stapler.

Figure A-3A

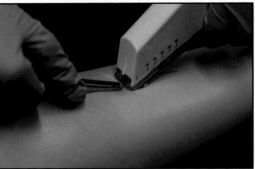

- Fully squeeze and then release the stapler handle or trigger to insert the staple in the skin.
- Lift the stapler from the wound and assess staple placement. The staple crossbar should be slightly elevated above the wound and periwound tissue (Figure A-3B).

Figure A-3B

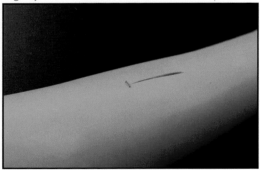

- Continue with the procedure until wound closure is complete.

Table A-8. Staple Removal on a Wound Model

- Position the 2-pronged lower jaw of the remover tool under the staple (Figure A-4A).

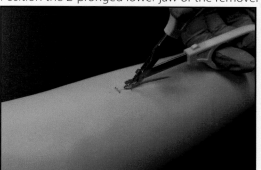

Figure A-4A

- Squeeze the handle of the remover tool until closed (Figure A-4B), bending the middle portion of the staple crossbar downward and the outer edges upward and lifting the staple from the tissues (Figure A-4C).

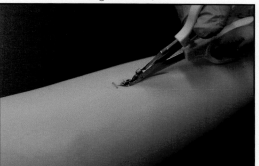

Figure A-4B

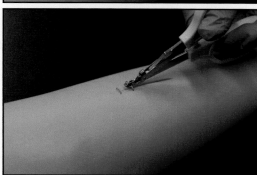

Figure A-4C

continued

Table A-8. Staple Removal on a Wound Model (continued)

- Keep the tool closed and move away from the wound with the staple engaged in the tool (Figure A-4D).

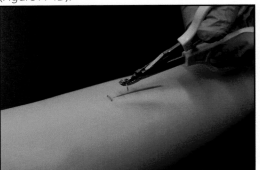

Figure A-4D

- Place each removed staple on gauze and count the total to ensure removal of all staples.

REFERENCES

1. Ediger MJ. Closure options for skin lacerations. *Int J Athl Ther Train.* 2010;15(2):19-22.
2. Forsch RT. Essentials of skin laceration repair. *Am Fam Physician.* 2008;78(8):945-951.
3. Honsik KA, Romeo MW, Hawley CJ, Romeo SJ, Romeo JP. Sideline skin and wound care for acute injuries. *Curr Sports Med Rep.* 2007;6(3):147-154.
4. Flanagan KW, Cuppett M. *Medical Conditions in the Athlete.* Human Kinetics; 2017:97-121.
5. Rose J, Tuma F. *Sutures and Needles.* StatPearls; 2021. Accessed June 17, 2022. https://www. ncbi.nlm.nih.gov/books/NBK539891/
6. Yag-Howard C. Sutures, needles, and tissue adhesives: A review for dermatologic surgery. *Dermatol Surg.* 2014;40(suppl 9):S3-S15.
7. Hochberg J, Meyer KM, Marion M. Suture choice and other methods of skin closure. *Surg Clin North Am.* 2009;89(3):627-641.
8. Hussey M, Bagg M. Principles of wound closure. *Oper Tech Sports Med.* 2011;19(4):206-211.
9. *Suturing 101: A stitch in time...* Provider Practice Essentials. Accessed June 20, 2022. https:// ppemedical.com/blog/suturing-101-a-stitch-in-time/
10. Dumville JC, Gray TA, Walter CJ, et al. Dressings for the prevention of surgical site infection. *Cochrane Database Syst Rev.* 2016;12:CD003091.
11. Copeland-Halperin LR, Via y Rada MLR, Levy J, Shank N, Funderburk CD, Shin JH. Does the timing of postoperative showering impact infection rates? A systematic review and meta-analysis. *J Plast Reconstr Aesthet Surg.* 2020;73(7):1306-1311.

B

WOUND CARE 101 INFOGRAPHIC

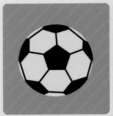
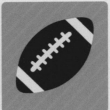
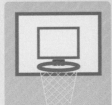
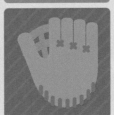

WOUND CARE 101

Injuries to the skin are common during athletic activities and proper management is important to promote healing and lessen the risk of infection. The management plan developed by the athletic trainer and the following recommendations can assist athletes/parents in the appropriate care of skin injuries.

DO

- Report all skin injuries to the athletic trainer as soon as possible.
- Practice good hand hygiene before and after cleaning and covering the wound.
    Wash hands with soap and water for at least 15 seconds and dry the hands with a disposable towel.
- Clean the wound and surrounding skin of all debris with tap water as soon as possible.
- Consider showering to clean larger wounds.
- Cover the wound with a dressing until fully healed.
- Change the dressing as instructed by the athletic trainer.
    Change sterile gauze, nonadherent pads, and adhesive strips and patches daily.
- Anticipate collection of fluid and/or swelling of modern moist dressings over the wound.

DON'T

- Scrub or soak the wound.
- Clean the wound daily.
- Use hydrogen peroxide or antiseptics to clean the wound.
- Remove the dressing unless instructed to by the athletic trainer.
- Change modern moist dressings (eg, films, blister bandages) daily.
- Let the wound breathe and dry out.

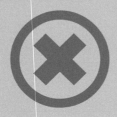

See the athletic trainer or other healthcare professional as soon as possible if pain, warmth, drainage, swelling, or redness increases; itching, rash, white discoloration, or fever develops; or healing does not occur.

Check in with the athletic trainer on a regular basis. You are encouraged to contact your athletic trainer with questions or for further information regarding wound care.

C

CLINICAL APPLICATION TABLE

Wound Type	Cleansing	Debridement	Dressing
Abrasion	*Wound bed:* Irrigation with normal saline or potable tap water at the appropriate temperature; showering with potable tap water at the appropriate temperature. *Periwound tissue:* Irrigation with normal saline or potable tap water; scrubbing with normal saline, potable tap water, or topical antiseptic.	Irrigation with normal saline or potable tap water; wet to moist; scrubbing with normal saline or potable tap water if heavily contaminated; conservative sharp;[a] autolytic with occlusive dressings	*Primary:* Occlusive (alginate, film, foam, hydrogel, and hydrocolloid), nonocclusive (woven or nonwoven sterile gauze, nonadherent pads, and adhesive strips and patches) based on wound, dressing, and patient factors. *Secondary:* Adhesive gauze or nonadherent, self-adherent, or adherent tapes and wraps based on wound, dressing, and patient factors.
Avulsion	*Wound bed:* Irrigation with normal saline or potable tap water. Do not use tap water if bone or tendon is exposed. *Avulsed tissue:* Gentle irrigation with normal saline.	Not indicated	*Primary:* Woven or nonwoven sterile gauze premoistened with normal saline. *Secondary:* Woven or nonwoven sterile gauze. *Avulsed tissue:* Woven or nonwoven sterile gauze premoistened with normal saline. Wrap the tissue and place it in a watertight bag. Place the bag in ice water or onto an ice bag, avoiding direct contact of the tissue with the ice. Refer the patient and avulsed tissue to a physician for further assessment and treatment.
Blister (closed, intact roof not impacting daily activities)	Not indicated	Not indicated	*Secondary:* Nonsterile hydrogel, nonocclusive (woven or nonwoven gauze, nonadherent pads, and adhesive strips and patches), adhesive gauze or nonadherent, self-adherent, or adherent tapes and wraps based on wound, dressing, and patient factors.

continued

Wound Type	Cleansing	Debridement	Dressing
Blister (closed, intact roof impacting daily activities)	*Blister roof and periwound tissue:* Scrubbing with topical antiseptic before debridement. *Wound bed:* Irrigation with normal saline or potable tap water after debridement.	*Blister roof:* Conservative sharp.[a] Create a small incision in the roof with a sterile, sharp instrument and drain fluid. Remove the roof by cutting along the border between the viable and nonviable tissue.	*Primary:* Occlusive (alginate, film, foam, hydrogel, and hydrocolloid), nonocclusive (woven or nonwoven sterile gauze, nonadherent pads, and adhesive strips and patches) based on wound, dressing, and patient factors. *Secondary:* Adhesive gauze or nonadherent, self-adherent, or adherent tapes and wraps based on wound, dressing, and patient factors.
Blister (open)	*Wound bed:* Irrigation with normal saline or potable tap water at the appropriate temperature. *Periwound tissue:* Irrigation with normal saline or potable tap water; scrubbing with normal saline, potable tap water, or topical antiseptic.	Irrigation with normal saline or potable tap water; wet to moist; scrubbing with normal saline or potable tap water if heavily contaminated; conservative sharp;[a] autolytic with occlusive dressings	*Primary:* Occlusive (alginate, film, foam, hydrogel, and hydrocolloid), nonocclusive (woven or nonwoven sterile gauze, nonadherent pads, and adhesive strips and patches) based on wound, dressing, and patient factors. *Secondary:* Adhesive gauze or nonadherent, self-adherent, or adherent tapes and wraps based on wound, dressing, and patient factors.

continued

Wound Type	Cleansing	Debridement	Dressing
Incision and laceration	*Wound bed:* Irrigation with normal saline or potable tap water. Do not use tap water if bone or tendon is exposed. *Periwound tissue:* Irrigation with normal saline or potable tap water; scrubbing with normal saline, potable tap water, or topical antiseptic.	Irrigation with normal saline or potable tap water. Do not use tap water if bone or tendon is exposed.	*Primary with adequate tissue approximation:* Occlusive (alginate, film, foam, hydrogel, and hydrocolloid), nonocclusive (woven or nonwoven sterile gauze, nonadherent pads, and adhesive strips and patches) based on the wound (superficial- to full-thickness), dressing, and patient factors. *Secondary:* Adhesive gauze or nonadherent, self-adherent, or adherent tapes and wraps based on wound, dressing, and patient factors. *Primary with tissue approximation required:* Dermal adhesives and wound closure strips based on the wound (minimal skin tension), dressing, and patient factors. *Secondary:* Woven or nonwoven sterile gauze, nonadherent pads, nonadherent or self-adherent wraps, and hypoallergenic skin tapes based on the wound, dressing, and patient factors. *Primary with tissue approximation required:* Sutures and staples based on the wound (high skin tension), dressing, and patient factors. *Secondary:* Woven or nonwoven sterile gauze, nonadherent pads, nonadherent or self-adherent wraps, and hypoallergenic skin tapes based on the wound, dressing, and patient factors. Possible referral to a physician for advanced cleansing, debridement, and wound closure.

continued

Wound Type	Cleansing	Debridement	Dressing
Puncture	*Wound bed:* Gentle irrigation with normal saline or potable tap water. *Periwound tissue:* Irrigation with normal saline or potable tap water; scrubbing with normal saline, potable tap water, or topical antiseptic	Consider the removal of visible, small objects with sterile instruments.[a] Use caution to avoid pushing objects deeper into the wound. Do not remove large or broken-off embedded objects from the wound.	*Primary with no cavity:* Occlusive (alginate, film, foam, hydrogel, and hydrocolloid), nonocclusive (woven or nonwoven sterile gauze, nonadherent pads, and adhesive strips and patches) based on the wound, dressing, and patient factors. *Secondary:* Adhesive gauze or nonadherent, self-adherent, or adherent tapes and wraps based on wound, dressing, and patient factors. *Primary with cavity:* Woven, nonwoven, and impregnated sterile gauze rolls and strips based on the wound, dressing, and patient factors. *Secondary:* Nonocclusive (woven or nonwoven sterile gauze, nonadherent pads, and adhesive strips and patches) based on wound, dressing, and patient factors. *Primary with embedded object:* Woven or nonwoven sterile gauze. Wrap gauze around the object, immobilize the object or joint, and refer to a physician for further assessment and treatment.

[a]Clinicians should review state laws and practice acts before performing this technique.

FINANCIAL DISCLOSURES

Dr. Joel W. Beam reported no financial or proprietary interest in the materials presented herein.

Dr. Bernadette Buckley reported no financial or proprietary interest in the materials presented herein.

Dr. Mario Ciocca reported no financial or proprietary interest in the materials presented herein.

INDEX

Note: Locators in *italic* indicate figures and in **bold** tables.

blisters 3–4, *4*, 53, *54*, 130, 139, **164–165**
bullae 114, 120, 143
bunching 89, *91*, 107, 130

CA-MRSA 114, 117
carbuncle 114, 117
cellulitis 114, *116*, 117, 120
Centers for Disease Control and Prevention 24
channels 73, *73*, **86**, 143
chemical burns 120
chemical debridement 58–59; contraindications 58; indications 58; procedures 59, *59*
clean technique 24–25, **25**, 26, 35, 144, 155, 157
cleaning 23–24, 143
cleansing 33–45; evidence 44–45; goal, purposes 34; patient, wound, clinician factors 34–35
cleansing solutions 41–44; normal saline 42, *42*, 44–45, 126–127; potable tap water 42, 44–45, 145; temperature 37, **38**, 41, 43–44, 126, 127
cleansing techniques 35–41, **164–167**; hydrotherapy 40–41; irrigation 35–37; scrubbing, swabbing 39–40, **164–167**; selection factors 34–35; showering 37, 44; supply and equipment **36**
clinical practice scenarios 125–142; adhered dressing removal for assessment 135; allergic contact dermatitis, diagnosing and treatment 136–137; dehiscence 137; delayed healing process, risk factor assessment 134; dressing removal, unauthorized, wound reassessment and education 127; dressing selection and transitions, lateral proximal thigh trauma, dressing options 128–129; education and adherence, wound care 133; erythematous maceration, development and treatment 129; eschar removal for assessment 132; medical product shortage, improvisation 126–127; MRSA transmission prevention 131; occlusive dressings choices for limited budgets 138–139, **139**; plantar foot blister treatment for aquatic activities 130; thenar eminence open blister, management plan 139–141
closure: primary 84, 145; secondary 84, 105, 130, 138, 145
community-associated methicillin-resistant *Staphylococcus aureus* (CA-MRSA) 114, 117
conservative sharp debridement 53–54; contraindications 53; indications 53; procedures 53–54, *54*
contamination 144; assessment 7, 35; cleaning and disinfection 23–24; cleansing 34, 35, 36, 39, 40, 41; debridement 55; dressings 65;

hand hygiene 16; PPE 23; sterile and clean techniques 24–25; wound management procedures 25–26; *see also* infection; infection control

debridement 49–60; efficacy, clinical evidence 59; goal, purposes 49–50; patient, wound, clinician factors 50; supply and equipment **51**
debridement, surgical 145, 148
debridement techniques 51–59, **164–167**; autolytic 51–52, *52*, 59; chemical 58–59, *59*; conservative sharp 53–54, *54*; hydrotherapy 57–58; irrigation 54–55; scrubbing 55–56, *55*; wet-to-moist 57; wet-to-dry 56–57
decontaminated 16, 23, 144
dehiscence **12**, 79, 117, 122, 137, 144
denuded 7, 106, 144
dermal adhesives **70**, 77–80, *78*, **83**, **86**, 89, **92–93**; advantages, disadvantages **83**, 117, 120, 122; application **92–93**; contraindications 78–79; evidence, clinical 79–80; indications 78, **83**; primary dressing 78, 89; wear duration **86**
dermis 1–2, *2*
desiccated **8**, 34, 52, 144
devitalized **8**, 53, *54*, 144
disinfection 23–24, 26, **36**, 144
dressing, selection and application 80–85; application and clinical pearls 93–97, *94–97*; application guidelines 85–93; dressing types characteristics **81–83**, 84–85; patient characteristics 85; wound characteristics 84; *see also* clinical practice scenarios; *dressings' own headings*
dressing types 65–79; nonocclusive 65–70, **66**, *67–69*, 79–80, **86**, 86–89, *87*, **88** *see also* nonocclusive dressings; occlusive **70**, 70–79, *71–75*, *77–78*, **82–83**, **86**, 89, 91–93, *91–95*, 95, *97 see also* occlusive dressings; selection, application 80, **81–83**, 84–85
dressings 63–97; adverse reactions 120; application guidelines 85–93; evidence, clinical 79–80; functions 65; moist wound healing 64; monitoring and reassessment 107; removal, unintended 127; selection, application, usage duration 80–85, **86**; types *see* dressing types; *individual dressings' headings*; wound dressings 63–64

ecchymosis 7, 106, 144
eczematous **12**, 144

Printed in the United States
by Baker & Taylor Publisher Services